FLUID BALANCE AND VOLUME RESUSCITATION FOR BEGINNERS

FLUID BALANCE AND VOLUME RESUSCITATION FOR BEGINNERS

GR Park MD DMedSci FRCA
Director of Intensive Care
and
Consultant in Anaesthesia

PG Roe BSc FRCA
Consultant in Anaesthesia
both at
Addenbrooke's Hospital, Cambridge

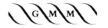

© 2000
Greenwich Medical Media Ltd
4th Floor
137 Euston Road
London
NW1 2AA

ISBN: 1 900151 545

First Published 2000
Reprinted 2001

Designed and Produced by
Diane Parker, Saldatore Limited

Printed in Great Britain by
The Alden Group, Oxford

Contents

The authors

K E Gunning, FRCS, FRCA   *Consultant in Anaesthesia*
                               and Intensive Care
M J Lindop, MA FRCA   *Consultant in Anaesthesia*
                               and Intensive Care
G R Park, MD DMedSci FRCA   *Director of Intensive Care*
                               and Consultant in Anaesthesia
P G Roe, BSc FRCA   *Consultant Anaesthetist*
R Ross Russell, MRCP   *Director of Paediatric*
                               Intensive Care

All at Addenbrooke's Hospital, Cambridge.

Preface

The topic of this book is important. Millions of patients throughout the world are given fluids, electrolytes and volume expanders every day. The choice of fluids is also huge. Their prescription is usually left to relatively junior doctors who often find the choice of fluid confusing, the electrolyte composition baffling and the amount they should give unclear. Many of the textbooks on the subject describe the physiology extremely well, but few will help the junior doctor solve a problem. This book will – we hope! It has been written by senior consultants, experts in their field, who not only know the theory, but also and perhaps more importantly deal with these problems every day. In addition, each of them trains junior doctors and so is aware of the problems they have.

To help trainees understand the problems with their topic we have asked each contributor to write in a didactic manner, using tables, diagrams, key points and bulleted lists to make their chapter easy to understand. The theory is there as well, but usually clearly separated to allow it to be read with the clinical part or delayed as the reader wishes. The first chapter deals with fundamental theory. This can be read later if wished. However, parts of the subsequent chapters may be less easy to understand if this course is taken.

This is not meant to be a comprehensive book on the topic – rather a practicable day to day guide. For example we have not included anything on the treatment of patients in renal failure. Readers of this book should obtain expert help in this and other problems not covered, rather than "dabble". Similarly, each chapter has a list of suggested further reading.

We hope you find this book of value. We would be pleased to receive comments from you (both good and bad) so that future editions can be improved.

Gilbert Park
Paul Roe
Cambridge
May 1999

Dedication

To the doctors, nurses and others we have had the privilege to teach over the years, their questioning minds have taught us much.

Abbreviations

δ	leakiness of a membrane
Π	osmotic pressure
κ	permeability of a membrane to water
ADH	antidiuretic hormone
AVP	arginine vasopressin
BP	blood pressure
Cl	chloride
CO	cardiac output
COP	colloid osmotic pressure
CVA	cerebrovascular accident
CVP	central venous pressure
Da	Dalton
DI	diabetes insipidus
DO_2	oxygen delivery
ECF	extracellular fluid
g	gram
h	hour
HAS	human albumin solution
Hb	haemoglobin
HES	hydroxyethyl starch
HMW	high molecular weight
HR	heart rate
ICF	intracellular fluid
ISF	interstitial fluid
iv	intravenous

K	potassium
kg	kilogram
L	litre
m	milli
min	minute
mol	mole
mv	micro vascular
MW	molecular weight
MW_n	number average molecular weight
MW_w	weight average molecular weight
MRI	magnetic resonance imaging
Na	sodium
NSAIDs	non steroidal anti-inflammatory drugs
osmol	osmoles
P	pressure
PAOP	pulmonary artery occlusion pressure
pmv	peri microvascular
$\dot{Q}$	net fluid flux
RES	reticulo endothelial system
Salt	sodium chloride
SIADH	syndrome of inappropriate secretion of anti-diuretic hormone
SIRS	systemic inflammatory response syndrome
SVR	systemic vascular resistance
TBW	total body water
TURP	transurethral resection of prostate

Normal fluid and electrolyte balance

There is often confusion about some of the terms used to describe fluid balance. The reader can choose; either refer to them when they crop up in the following chapters or read them now. Whatever, their understanding is essential.

Total body water

- In a 70 kg man, total body water (TBW) is approximately 42 L which is 60% of total body weight.
- In females this is reduced to 50% of total body weight as there is more fat which contains less water.
- In infants with very little fat, TBW is greater than 60% of total body weight.
- The elderly have a reduction in TBW to less than 50% of total body mass as muscle mass (with high water content) decreases with age.
- TBW can be divided into intracellular and extracellular compartments (Figure 1). The extracellular compartment can be further divided into interstitial and intravascular compartments.

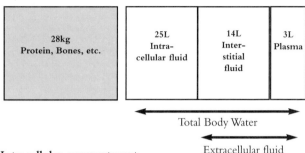

Intracellular compartment

Extracellular fluid

Figure 1: The different body fluid compartments in a 70 kg man.

- This contains intracellular fluid (ICF).
- The ICF has a volume of 25 litres.
- Its principal cation is potassium and as it contains twice the number of osmotic particles as the extracellular fluid (ECF); it has twice the volume.

- The cell membrane is impermeable to electrolytes which therefore contribute to the osmotic forces here. Because ICF and ECF are isotonic, there is osmotic equilibrium at the cell membrane.

- The ICF volume is sensitive to changes in the sodium con-centration of the ECF because a high serum or ECF sodium concentration will result in movement of water out of the cells by osmosis. The reverse occurs with a low serum sodium.
- As potassium is predominantly intracellular, serum potassium is a poor measure of total body potassium.

Extracellular compartment
- The size of the extracellular compartment is determined by homeostatic control of both its tonicity and volume.
- Alterations in tonicity, detected at osmoreceptors in the brain, affect both thirst and levels of arginine vasopressin (AVP) altering both the intake and output of water.
- Altered ECF volume can be detected by volume receptors in the circulation. These are found in the large veins and right atrium.
- The kidney also controls ECF volume. A reduction in systemic arterial pressure reduces renal perfusion pressure leading to an increase in renin secretion from the juxtaglomerular apparatus

resulting in angiotensin II and aldosterone release (Page 108). This causes sodium and water retention.

• The total amount (not concentration) of sodium in the ECF determines its volume and consequently, homeostatic mechanisms controlling volume are mainly concerned with the retention or excretion of sodium (Chapter 2). If a sodium load is added to the ECF such that tonicity increases, thirst will be stimulated and water retention by the kidneys will occur.

The ECF volume therefore increases and this stimulates a loss of sodium (with water) which eventually returns the ECF volume to normal.

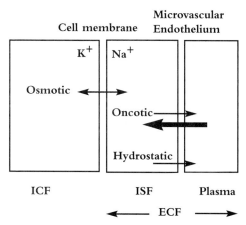

Figure 2: The three fluid compartments. The ICF and ISF (interstitial fluid) are separated by the cell membrane. The ISF and the plasma are separated by the microvascular endothelium.

Molarity
A mole of a substance is its molecular weight expressed in grams. The molarity of a solution is the number of moles dissolved in one litre of solvent. Molality is the number of moles dissolved in 1000 g of solvent.

Flux
This term describes the process of flow of a substance from one place to another.

Osmosis
A membrane is semi-permeable if it allows free passage of small molecules (solvent – for example, water), but not of larger molecules (solute – for example, protein). If the large molecules are restricted to one side of the membrane, they reduce the concentration of small molecules on this side by occupying space. The concentration of small molecules will thus be greater on the other side and will diffuse along their concentration gradient. The pressure required to counter this effect is the osmotic pressure.

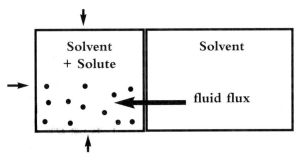

Figure 3: Osmotic pressure. Solute occupies space on one side of a semipermeable membrane. This reduces the concentration of solvent on this side of the membrane. Solvent then flows down its concentration gradient (flux). The osmotic pressure is the pressure that would be required to stop this flux (represented as the small arrows).

Osmolality
An osmole is a mole of substance multiplied by the number of particles it forms in solution. Sodium chloride, theoretically an 'ideal' solution, dissociates into two ions (sodium and chloride) and therefore one mmol gives rise to two mosmol. However, the effect of producing two particles by sodium chloride is reduced by both incomplete ionisation and ionic interactions in plasma which is not an 'ideal' solvent. This results in one mmol of sodium chloride producing 1.86 mosmol.

Plasma osmolality is a measure of the total number of particles in a given weight of plasma.

The difference between osmolarity and osmolality.

- The osmolarity of a solution is the number of moles of solute dissolved in one litre of solvent.
- The osmolality of a solution is the number of moles of solute dissolved in one kilogram of solvent.

There is little difference between the two, but osmolality is preferred as it is independent of the small volume changes which occur when a fluid changes temperature.

Osmolality and osmotic pressure are quite different. It is important to appreciate that the osmolality of a solution refers to the total number of particles in a given weight of solvent *in-vitro*. *In-vivo*, at a biological membrane, the osmotic pressure developed will depend upon which solutes the membrane is impermeable to. For example, at vascular endothelium, electrolytes (which contribute a large part of the osmolality of plasma) do not in isolation result in osmotic pressure as this membrane is permeable to them. However, the vascular endothelium is impermeable to plasma proteins. Although they contribute only a very small part of the total osmolality of plasma (because there are only a small number of protein particles compared to ionic particles), they are the main providers of the osmotic pressure at this membrane.

Tonicity

Substances which are restricted to the ECF, principally sodium and its associated anions chloride and bicarbonate, are important in determining the volume of this compartment and are said to provide 'effective osmoles'. The concentration of effective osmoles is known as the tonicity. Substances such as urea pass into cells and therefore do not provide effective osmoles, although they do contribute to the osmolality of plasma. Glucose does provide effective osmoles as long as it remains in the plasma. An isotonic solution does not result in a net movement of water in and out of cells when given intravenously because there is no change in the osmolality of the ECF and therefore no change in the osmotic pressure at the cell membrane.

Colloid osmotic pressure

The term colloid refers to large gelatinous molecules with molecular weights in excess of an arbitrary figure of 10,000 Dalton, for example, plasma proteins. If a semipermeable membrane restrains the passage of these molecules, but allows ionic salts to pass, the osmotic pressure developed by these colloid molecules is the colloid osmotic pressure (COP).

Oncotic pressure

This is often used synonymously with colloid osmotic pressure, but there is a distinct difference. Oncotic pressure is the osmotic pressure developed at the vascular endothelium by whatever means. It results in large part from the plasma proteins (COP); also osmotic effects of electrolytes held in the plasma by the negatively charged proteins (Gibbs–Donnan effect) contribute.

Gibbs–Donnan equilibrium

In a two compartment system, the product of the concentration of diffusable ions in one compartment will equal the product of the same ions in the other compartment with the total cationic and anionic charges being equal in each compartment. However, the distribution of diffusable ions across the semipermeable membrane will be unequal if a poorly diffusable ion is present with an unequal distribution. Plasma has such a poorly diffusable anion (albumin, charge - 17) and this results in a greater number of diffusable cations (sodium) in this compartment (see Figure 4C).

The cell membrane

Fluid fluxes at this membrane are determined by osmosis. The cell membrane is semipermeable. Water passes through freely, but electrolytes do not. A high intracellular concentration of potassium is maintained by energy dependent active transport mechanisms. Apart from situations of chronic total body potassium depletion, the intracellular osmolarity usually remains constant. Fluid fluxes at this membrane therefore arise as a result of changes in ECF sodium concentration. Hypernatraemia results in a reduced ECF volume. Hyponatraemia results in an increased ICF volume.

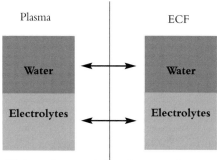

A. Equilibrium of water and electrolytes (in isolation) at the microvascular membrane

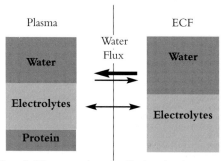

B: Effect of adding an uncharged colloid to the plasma (Colloid osmotic pressure)

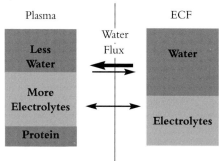

C: Effect of taking into account the negative charge on the protein (Gibbs Donnan effect)

Figure 4: A,B,C summarising the effects of the water movement, the effects of colloid osmotic pressure and the Gibbs Donnan effect.

The microvascular endothelium

The intravascular and extracellular compartments are separated by the microvascular endothelium which is freely permeable to water and electrolytes, but is relatively impermeable to proteins.

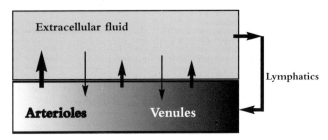

Figure 5: Fluid fluxes at the microvascular membrane. Fluid moves out of the microvasculature as a result of hydrostatic pressure. This is greater in the arterioles than in the venules. Fluid moves back into the microvasculature as a result of oncotic pressure. There is also a movement of fluid from the ECF back into the circulation via the lymphatics, thus bypassing the microvascular membrane.

Fluid fluxes at this membrane can be described by the Starling-Landis equation:

$$\dot{Q} = \kappa \, [(P_{mv} - P_{pmv}) - \sigma \, (\Pi_{mv} - \Pi_{pmv})]$$

or

$$\dot{Q} = \kappa \, \Delta P - \sigma \, \Delta \, \Pi$$

Where

$\dot{Q}$ is the net fluid flux
P is hydrostatic pressure
Π is osmotic pressure

Microvascular (mv) refers to the environment within the capillaries in the tissues.

Perimicrovascular (pmv) refers to the environment immediately outside of these vessels and in equilibrium with them.

κ is how permeable the membrane is to water (the hydraulic conductivity).

σ is an indication of how leaky (semipermeable) the membrane is (reflection coefficient). If σ is less than 1, solute (protein) will to some extent pass through the membrane. This means there will be a fractional reduction in the osmotic pressure generated by a given concentration of protein on one side of the membrane.

It is important to appreciate that the protein concentration of interstitial fluid is 20 – 40% (70% in the lung) less than that of plasma. With a reflection coefficient (leakiness) of 0.8 in health, the contribution of osmosis to opposing fluid egress is small. Consequently, there is a net flux of fluid and protein out of the vascular compartment into the interstitial compartment.

This excess fluid is taken up by lymphatics which have a total flow of 1-3 L per day. This has the capacity to increase greatly, preventing oedema formation.

The interstitial compartment

The interstitial compartment contains 33% of the total body water. It has important transport functions between plasma and cells. There are two subcompartments, parenchymal (perimicrovascular) and loose binding connective tissue. Fluid filtered from the plasma passes into the perimicrovascular compartment, which contains functional space between vessels and cells, and is immediately taken up by the lymphatics which act as an overflow for small increases in pressure and volume. In health these lymphatics have a high capacity. If the capacity of lymphatic drainage is exceeded, it first overflows into the loose binding connective tissue which is normally dry. Lymphatics are unable to remove excess interstitial fluid from the loose binding connective tissue which has a high capacity. Accumulation of fluid in the loose, binding connective tissue results in oedema. This fluid no longer has the normal physiological function of interstitial fluid and is temporarily 'lost'. It has been referred to as the 'third space' and remains in place until reabsorbed into the vasculature. If the volume of this space is exceeded, it may overflow out of the tissues into body cavities, for example as pleural effusions, ascites and into the alveolii as pulmonary oedema.

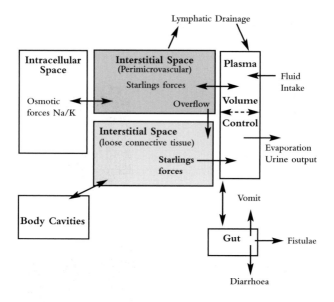

Figure 6: The two subcompartments of the interstitial fluid and how they relate to other body fluid compartments.

The interstitial compartment in the lung

In the normal lung, a reduced colloid osmotic pressure results in an increased fluid flux from the plasma to the interstitial compartment. Normally this will not result in an increase in extravascular lung water because of the high capacity of the lymphatic drainage. However, when fluid movement into the perimicrovascular space of the lung exceeds the capacity of lymphatic drainage, pulmonary oedema occurs. Initially, this fluid is confined to the distensible interstitial space which occurs between layers of loose alveolar epithelium away from the pulmonary capillary. The closely applied capillary endothelium and alveolar epithelium, which is the principal site of gas exchange, is largely spared at this stage and consequently there is little effect on gas exchange. As extravascular lung water increases, further interstitial distension occurs, and fluid begins to leak out into the alveoli. In the alveoli, hydrophobic surfactant creates forces which minimise this leakage, but eventually alveolar flooding occurs (pulmonary oedema). It is only at this stage that a significant impairment of gas exchange occurs.

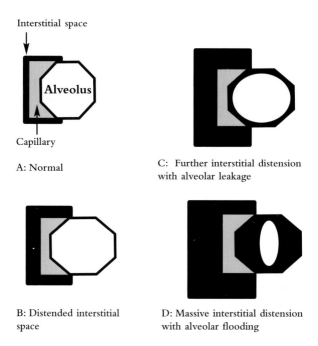

A: Normal

C: Further interstitial distension with alveolar leakage

B: Distended interstitial space

D: Massive interstitial distension with alveolar flooding

Figure 7: The four stages of pulmonary oedema.

Renal threshold

The glomerulus has "pores" that allow molecules to pass through. The size of the substance allowed to pass through will depend on both its molecular weight and shape. Thus, substances will be filtered through the glomerulus when their molecular weight is below a certain threshold value. As different substances have molecules of different shape, the value of this threshold will vary with the substance. In addition, the charge of a molecule will also affect renal filtration as the glomerular basement membrane has a negative charge. This explains the low filtration from plasma of albumin, which has a negative charge and is therefore repelled.

Abnormalities of salt and water balance

Changes in electrolyte and water balance are common. They are frequently mistreated. Careful examination of the patient and interpretation of the results will prevent this. Both abnormalities of sodium and water balance will be reflected in the serum concentration of sodium. When salt is mentioned in this book the meaning is sodium chloride. The normal range for serum concentration of sodium in our laboratory is 135-145 mmol/L. It may differ slightly in other laboratories. Some of the common causes of salt and water abnormalities are shown in Table 1.

Abnormalities of sodium balance

These are primarily a result of a deficit or an excess of salt and result in changes in the volume, but not necessarily the tonicity of the ECF. The concentration of sodium in the plasma indicates the amount of water relative to the amount of sodium. Hypernatraemia results in contracted ICF volume and hyponatraemia results in an expanded ICF volume.

Salt deficit
A primary deficit of salt is usually a result of increased loss of either salt alone or salt and water with water replacement. It may occur with diarrhoea, Addison's disease, diabetic ketoacidosis, with ascites and in cases of chronic renal failure. Salt deficiency results in an early reduction in the volume of the ECF, and consequently the circulating blood volume, with haemoconcentration and an increased blood urea. Intracellular dehydration does not occur. The clinical picture is of early circulatory failure. It is important to appreciate that it is the total amount of salt in the ECF which is of

Water deficit

- Reduced intake (inability to drink)
- Diabetes insipidus

Water excess

- Administration of IV free water
- TUR syndrome

Sodium deficit

- Diarrhoea
- Addison's disease
- Diabetic ketoacidosis
- Ascites
- Chronic renal failure

Sodium excess

- 8.4% NaHCO$_3$
- Seawater ingestion
- Treatment of ketoacidosis with 0.9% saline.

Table 1: Some of the commoner causes of salt and water abnormalities.

importance here. There may be little change in the serum sodium concentration. Sodium deficiency leads to water loss as a compensatory mechanism, whereas sodium excess leads to water retention and oedema. Salt deficiency is treated with 0.9% sodium chloride and losses may be up to ten litres, although considerable circulatory disturbance will occur with losses in excess of four litres.

Changes in blood pressure and pulse are late signs and visual impressions of perfusion and hydration (skin turgor) are non-specific and difficult to quantify as signs of hypovolaemia. The use of central venous monitoring should be undertaken when in doubt (Page 51), although this is insensitive with relatively large changes being required to show an effect. Where hypovolaemia is suspected it is important to assess the response of the patient to repeated fluid boluses (Page 55) rather than to consider a single set of signs or values. Over a timescale of days, mesurement of serial patient weights is an invaluable aid to the assessment of overall fluid balance.

Salt excess

Salt excess may occur in the following circumstances:

- Administration of 8.4% $NaHCO_3$.
- Ingestion of seawater
- Administration of 0.9% saline in large volumes to the patient where the losses are hypotonic e.g. diabetes mellitus.

The ECF is expanded.

Hypernatraemia is rarely a result of a net gain in sodium.

> Hypernatraemia results in cell shrinkage
> Hyponatraemia results in cell swelling

The patient with a high sodium

The serum sodium is greater than 145 mmol/L. The usual cause of hypernatraemia is water loss. This can be renal loss associated with loss of weight, but may also be caused by gastrointestinal or other losses.

What to look for

- Is the heart rate increased and blood pressure reduced?
  If so, the intracellular volume is contracted. The patient is salt and water depleted.

- What is the urine osmolality?
  It should be maximal (1300 mOsm/kg and with low urine volume if there is water and salt depletion. If the urine osmolarity is low, is the patient on diuretics? If the urine osmolarity is very low consider diabetes insipidus (DI). There is a lack of antidiuretic hormone (ADH) if the pituitary is damaged. In certain types of kidney damage "nephrogenic DI" may occur. Nephrogenic and central types may be distinguished by the response of a dose of ADH (Page 20).

- Is there extracellular fluid volume expansion as evidenced by oedema, increased jugular venous pressure and weight gain? If so then an excess of salt is likely although this is not a common cause of hypernatraemia.

Treatment of hypernatraemia

Stop losses of water

Stop diuretics, reduce gastro-intestinal losses with anti-diarrhoeal agents if appropriate (see Table 2), give antidiuretic hormone if there is central diabetes insipidus.

Appropriate	Inappropriate
Travellers diahorrea	Villous adenoma
Enteral feed intolerance	Spurious diarrhoea
	Clostridium diffcle infection
	Active ulcerative colitis

Table 2: Some causes of diarrhoea where anti-diarrhoeal treatment should and should not be used.

Replace water
The deficit should be replaced slowly preferably by the oral route. Aim to correct serum sodium by no more than 12 mmol/L over 24 hrs. If the patient is asymptomatic there is even less urgency to treatment. If the patient is convulsing, it is necessary to reduce the sodium urgently, for example, by 6 mmol/L over one hour. This can be achieved by intravenous infusion of 5% glucose solution with regular serum estimations of sodium in a high dependency environment.

When hypernatremia is a result of excessive sodium administration a diuretic is used to promote the loss of sodium and water. Water is given by mouth if possible or intravenously as 5% glucose solution.

The patient with a low sodium
The serum sodium concentration is less than 135 mmol/L. Usually hyponatraemia is a result of excess water. However, if the extra-cellular fluid volume is depleted (see below) then there must also be a loss of total body sodium although this is much less common.

What to look for
- What is the serum osmolarity?
  It should be low. Whenever you measure this always check the result by roughly calculating the serum osmolarity from the following equation:
  Serum osmolarity = (2 × [Na + K]) + urea + glucose) (units in mmol/L) If the measured and calculated disagree by about 10 mOsm/kg consider pseudohypernatraemia (see below) or hyperglycaemia.

- Is there ECF volume depletion? Is there a loss of weight, absence of oedema, loss of skin turgor, low CVP?
  If so, there is a loss of total body sodium and this will need to be replaced.
- Is the patient symptomatic (nausea, headache, confusion, seizures – signs of brain cell swelling)?
  If so, then treatment will need to be more rapid initially. If the patient is asymptomatic, then treatment will be slow. Symptoms usually occur in acute hyponatraemia. It is not always possible to know how rapidly hyponatraemia has developed when the patient presents.

How fast to treat

Slow treatment in the asymptomatic patient

Increase the serum sodium concentration at a rate of no more than 0.5 mmol/l/h (12 mmol/day) in the first 24h. Thereafter, treatment may be slower. It is not necessary to increase the serum sodium higher than 125 – 130 mmol/L.

Faster treatment in the symptomatic patient

> Symptomatic hyponatraemia is a medical emergency which needs urgent and closely monitored treatment.

If the patient is convulsing, the sodium may be increased by 6 mmol/L in the first hour. For lesser symptoms, rapid correction may be slower than this but should stop either after the sodium has been increased by 6 mmol/L or when symptoms stop whichever is sooner. Therafter, correction should be at a rate of 0.5 mmol/L/h. The maximum change should be 18 mmol/L in the first 24 hrs.

> There is a risk of developing central pontine myelinolysis if correction of hyponatremia is too rapid.

Central pontine myelinolysis is a complication of rapid correction of chronic hyponatraemia. There is destruction of medullary sheaths in the centre of the basilar portion of the pons. It has wide variations in the clinical features which range from coma and flaccid quadriplegia to minor behavioral changes. The clinical effects of CPM may take several days to develop and may need a MRI to confirm the diagnosis.

Acute hyponatraemia of less than three days duration is usually iatrogenic. Treatment may proceed more rapidly and an increase in the serum sodium level of 24 mmol/L/day is acceptable. 0.9% sodium chloride is given and diuretics are used to excrete the water excess. Hypertonic sodium chloride solutions have been used, not because sodium is deficient, but to increase plasma tonicity and reduce the development of cerebral oedema. Complications of acute restoration of serum sodium levels are of fluid overload (increased ECF volume) secondary to excessive sodium administration.

How to treat hyponatraemia

The patient with hypotonic hyponatraemia without ECF volume depletion
- The problem is water excess.
- If the patient is asymptomatic, treatment may be slow and is achieved by water restriction.
- If the patient is symptomatic, water restriction alone will not achieve the desired rate of increase in serum sodium. Small volumes of hypertonic saline may be given (e.g.100 mL of 1.8% saline) with repeated estimations of serum sodium. If the patient is oedematous, then it is clear that there is an increase in the ECF volume.In this case, giving extra sodium ions will only increase this further and it will be necessary to consider active measures to increase water loss. Furosemide or mannitol may be given, but urinary sodium should be measured and replaced.In some refractory patients, such as those with liver disease, continuous veno-venous haemofiltration may need to be used.

The patient with hypotonic hyponatraemia and a contracted ECF volume
- The problem is sodium depletion.
- If the patient is asymptomatic, treatment may be slow and is achieved by the administration of 0.9% sodium chloride solution.
- If the patient is symptomatic, the desired rate of increase in serum sodium is achieved with either 0.9% saline or 1.8% saline.
- Regardless of symptoms, it may be necessary to infuse fluids rapidly to resuscitate the low ECF volume. In this case it is important to use fluids which are isotonic to the patient or sudden dangerous changes in the serum concentration of sodium may result.

Changes in water balance

These are primarily a result of a deficiency or an excess of water and result in changes in the tonicity, but not necessarily the volume of the ECF.

Water deficit

A primary deficit of water is commonly the result of a reduced intake, secondary to an inability to drink. Increased losses may also occur in central and nephrogenic diabetes insipidus. Water deficiency results in cellular dehydration as a result of increased ECF tonicity.

Plasma volume remains normal until late. Water deficit is the commonest cause of hypernatraemia. Treatment is with 5% glucose solutions, although care is needed if hypernatraemia is present as rapid rehydration will lead to cerebral oedema. Deficits may be up to ten litres.

Some of the changes in salt and water balance are summarised in Table 3.

	Serum Sodium	HR	Blood pressure	Oedema	Urine osmol	Urine Sodium
Condition Sodium overload	↑	N(↑)	N(↑)	++	↑+	↑
Water depletion	↑	↑	↓	–	↑++	↓
Water overload	↓	N(↑)	N(↑)	Acute– chronic ↓	↓ N(↓)	N
Sodium depletion	↓	↑	↓	–	↓	↓

Table 3: Summary of changes in salt and water balance.
↑ increased, ↓ decreased, N normal, ( ) occasionally,
  – absent, + present.

Water excess

Water excess (increased TBW) is most commonly a result of administration of free water (5% glucose, 4% glucose/0.18% sodium chloride or 1.5% glycine irrigation during transurethral surgery - see below). It causes hyponatraemia which is rarely a result of sodium loss. Hyponatraemia may also occur with the syndrome of inappropriate antidiuretic hormone secretion (SIADH) which occurs with certain tumours, central nervous system disorders and pulmonary sepsis. Excessive ADH secretion also occurs in the perioperative period.

TURP Syndrome

Patients undergoing transurethral resection of prostate (TURP) will have large volume bladder irrigation with a non-electrolyte solution (glycine). 0.9% saline cannot be used during electrosurgery as it would disperse the current. A large volume of glycine solution can be absorbed by the exposed veins in the prostatic bed. This will result in quite marked hyponatraemia with an expanded ECF (oedema). The glycine will act as a particle in the ECF and may result in movement of water out of cells (as seen in hypernatraemia). Consequently, there will be less cell swelling than in a hyponatraemia of this degree that is simply a result of a gain in free water. Measured serum osmolality will be greater than the calculated one - confirming the presence of the new particle (glycine). In the absence of cerebral symptoms, the patient should be allowed to excrete the glycine and extra water. Glycine is an osmotic diuretic and Na^+ will be lost. This will need to be replaced to keep the ECF volume normal.

Polydipsia in mental disease

There is usually a psychiatric history. Water is ingested to excess and a dilute urine is produced. If there is insufficient osmolar intake, sodium will be lost in the urine. A decrease in ECF volume will occur, resulting in an excretion of ADH which will reduce the urine output. In addition to sodium loss, there is then also water retention.

Syndrome of inappropriate secretion of antidiuretic hormone (SIADH)

This is a result of the presence of antidiuretic hormone (ADH) - also known as vasopressin - which is not a result of its two physiological stimuli – hypernatraemia and low effective circulatory volume (Table 4). This will result in a hyponatraemic patient with a high effective circulating volume. The inappropriate ADH may arise from the posterior pituitary or from a neoplasm. (See also Page 107 for a description of the importance of vasopressin after surgery.)

Syndrome of Inappropriate Anti Diuretic Hormone Secretion	Central causes of diabetes insipidus
Tumours (oat cell Ca lung) Drugs: NSAIDs, phosphodiesterase inhibitors Perioperative stress CNS lesions	Head trauma and neuro-surgery Intracranial neoplasm Central infections Hypoxia CVA Drugs

Table 4: Abnormalities of vasopressin excretion.

Pseudohyponatremia
Serum contains 93% water. The remainder consists of lipids, proteins and salts. In hyperlipidaemia and hyperproteinaemia, the amount of water in serum will be reduced, and this will alter the serum sodium assay, even though the ratio of sodium to water will be normal and the serum osmolality will be normal. This is called pseudohyponatremia. It does not require treatment as osmotic forces at the cell membrane are unchanged.

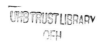

Crystalloids

Fluids are normally drunk each day to supply the normal requirements of water. If fluids cannot be taken orally or by nasogastric tube they are usually given intravenously.

Maintenance fluids are calculated according to the following formula: 4 mL/kg/h for the first 10 kg of body weight, 2 mL/kg/h for the second 10 kg and 1 mL/kg/h thereafter (Table 5). For most adult patients 3 L/day is adequate.

Patient Weight (kg)	mL/hr	mL/day
50	90	2169
60	100	2400
70	110	2640
80	120	2880
90	130	3120
100	140	3360

Table 5: Maintenance fluid volumes for differing patient weights.

When calculating the maintenance fluid needs for a patient it is important to take into account the additional fluids being given with drugs and nutrition. Failure to do this may result in fluid overload. In addition to fluids, the body also needs a minimum amount of electrolytes to replace its losses.

The daily requirements of electrolytes are 50-150 mmol of sodium and 20-40 mmol of potassium. This may be achieved by infusion of 4% glucose/0.18% sodium chloride solution (3 litres in 24 hrs) which provides 93 mmol sodium or 1 litre of 0.9% sodium chloride followed by two litres of 5% glucose (3 litres in 24 hrs) which provides 154 mmol of sodium. Potassium is added after 24 hrs as guided by serum estimations.

(See also Chapter 8 for managing surgical patients.)

> If there is renal dysfunction the amount of fluid and electrolytes needed will be changed - probably reduced.

Hypovolaemia

> Hypovolaemia is a medical emergency

When fluid is lost from the body, the three body fluid compartments (intracellular, interstitial and plasma) may each be depleted and require separate consideration. All may be affected in different ways in different situations. The distinction between extracellular and plasma depletion is difficult clinically and leads to some disagreements as to treatment. The key objective in fluid resuscitation is to restore the circulating plasma volume to normal as rapidly as possible. (Chapter 5).

Intracellular compartment
Intracellular depletion occurs with dehydration and hypernatraemia (which is almost always a result of water loss). Water may be replaced with 5% glucose solution, but see also Chapter 2 on patients with high sodium.

Plasma and interstitial compartments
Crystalloid solutions containing iso-osmotic amounts of sodium (i.e. 0.9% sodium chloride) are distributed throughout the extracellular compartment (plasma and interstitial space) and therefore

resuscitate both spaces. Colloids are confined initially to the plasma (although some are more efficient in this regard). Both may be given to resuscitate a low circulating blood volume.

> If crystalloids are given to resuscitate a patient, about three times the amount will be required than if colloids are given because of the difference in distribution.

THEORY

What are crystalloids and what different types are available

Crystalloids are solutions of ions (Na^+ & Cl^-) and/or small sugars (glucose) in water. They are cheap to make, unlike colloids. Most are approximately isoosmotic with plasma (see Table 6). They pass freely through the microvascular endothelium and do not, by themselves, contribute to oncotic pressure. After intravenous administration, the distribution of these fluids is determined by their sodium concentration. As sodium is largely restricted to the extracellular compartment, solutions containing isotonic concentrations of this ion will distribute through the whole of this compartment. Solutions containing less sodium, and whose osmotic activity is maintained with glucose, effectively contain water only (since the glucose is metabolised) which is able to distribute into the intracellular compartment (see Figure 1). The amount of 'free water' in a crystalloid preparation is determined by its sodium content with respect to 0.9% normal saline. 1000 mL of a 5% glucose solution contains 1000 mL of free water and will be distributed evenly throughout the total body water. 0.9% sodium chloride solution contains no free water and will be restricted to the extracellular compartment. 1000 ml of 4% glucose/0.18% sodium chloride contains 30 mmol of sodium which is 1/5 of that of 0.9% saline. 1/5 of the litre (200 mL) may be considered to be 0.9% saline and the remaining 4/5 (800 mL) to be free water.

0.9% sodium chloride
This solution contains 154 mmol/L of both sodium and chloride ions and is isotonic with serum. It is used as a volume expander and to treat sodium depletion. 154 mmol is, however, well above the daily requirement and sodium overload (with increased ECF volume) may result from indiscriminate use of this product in the

absence of a sodium deficit. It is primarily distributed in the extra-cellular compartment. It may be used for volume resuscitation in crystalloid based regimens, but has the potential to produce hyper-chloraemic acidosis, when used in large volumes, particularly in patients with renal impairment. As with balanced electrolyte solutions (see below), administration of three times the volume of blood loss is required to replace plasma volume.

Balanced electrolyte solutions

These solutions are isotonic and contain potassium and calcium in addition to sodium and chloride ions. Certain brands also contain lactate which is metabolised to bicarbonate. It is important to appreciate that this bicarbonate is not immediately available. The purpose of these solutions is to maintain the composition of the extracellular environment when large volumes of intravenous fluids are required over a short period of time. They form the basis of volume resuscitation in the crystalloid based regimens which are standard in the United States and in advanced trauma life support (ATLS) protocols. They are also useful in the intraoperative period when several litres of fluid may need to be given rapidly. In the US, a preparation of Ringers lactate is available with 50 g of glucose per litre; 5% glucose in Ringers lactate. This is a hyperosmotic solution. It does not contain free water.

5% glucose

This is essentially water. The glucose is added simply to render it isoosmotic, although its calorific value may be exploited. Glucose solutions contain the dextro (δ-) isomer of glucose. Glucose contributes to the tonicity of plasma, but this is short lived in the presence of insulin when it is rapidly taken up by cells. The water is then distributed throughout the TBW and produces negligible plasma volume expansion. Severe hyponatraemia will result if this product is infused rapidly. It is usually administered slowly, alternating with 0.9% saline for maintenance therapy.

5% glucose should not be used to treat hypotension or oliguria If 1000 mL of 5% glucose is given only (5/50 × 1000) = 100 mL will remain in the circulation.

	Na$^+$ (mmol/L)	Cl$^-$ (mmol/L)	K$^+$ (mmol/L)	Mg^{2+} (mmol/L)	Ca^{2+} (mmol/L)	Gluconate (mmol/L)	HCO$_3^-$ (mmol/L)	Glucose (g/dL)	Calculated Osmolality (mosmol/L)
Serum values	142	103	4.5	0.9	2.5	–	26	0.1	290
0.9% sodium chloride	154(150)	154(150)	–	–	–	–	–	–	308
5% glucose								5	278
4% glucose/0.18% sodium chloride	31(30)	31(30)	–	–	–	–	–	4	284
Hartmann's solution	131	111	5	–	2	–	29 (as lactate)	–	278
Lactated Ringer's solution (US)	130	109	4	–	1.5	–	28		273
Ringer's solution for injection (UK)	147	156	4	–	2.2	–	–	–	311
Plasmalyte 148	140	98	5	1.5	–	23	–	–	296
Plasmalyte M	40	40	16	91.5	2.5	23	12	5	406

Table 6: Electrolyte concentrations of normal serum and common crystalloid solutions.

Glucose-saline solutions

A variety of mixtures of glucose and saline are available with considerable international variation. Depending on the precise mixture, these solutions can be considered to be a mixture of 0.9% saline and free water. The most commonly employed mixture in the UK is 4% glucose/0.18% sodium chloride ("dextrose saline") which is isotonic. This may be used as a maintenance fluid at a rate of 2-3 litres per day in an adult. Care is needed in the perioperative period when both sodium and water are retained. As 1000 mL of this product only contains 30 mmol of sodium, dilutional hyponatraemia may result. In the US, mixtures of 5% glucose with 0.45% sodium chloride and 5% glucose with 0.9% sodium chloride are common and avoid the problem of hyponatraemia encountered with 4% glucose/0.18% sodium chloride. These solutions are, however, hyperosmotic. One litre of 5% glucose with 0.45% sodium chloride contains 500 mL of free water. One litre of 5% glucose with 0.9% sodium chloride contains no free water.

Colloids

Colloids are solutions of large molecules with molecular weights of greater than 10,000 Daltons (Da). They contribute to the oncotic pressure at the microvascular endothelium. Unlike crystalloids, they are initially confined to the plasma and will produce a greater expansion of this compartment than crystalloids. It is important to appreciate that this effect is temporary with all colloids and a wide variation in efficacy between different types exists. For example, gelatins have a duration of action of 1-4h, whereas starches may act for 4 to 24h. Some colloid preparations, for example 20% albumin, have a greater oncotic pressure than plasma and in normal humans tend to draw water into the plasma (plasma expanders) at the expense of the interstitial space.

There are four major types of colloids, albumin, gelatins, dextrans and starches.

Albumin

Human albumin solution (HAS) is derived from pooled human serum. Its advantages compared to other colloids and as a treament for hypoalbuminaemia have been questioned for some time. More recently further doubt has been cast on its use by the publication of a meta analysis. This was based on old studies and suggested that its use was associated with an increased mortality. However, the consensus view of the subsequent correspondence provoked by this paper was that further studies are needed in carefully controlled trials.

Albumin has a molecular weight of 69,000 Da. It is the primary oncotic particle in the plasma accounting for 70 - 80% of oncotic pressure in normal humans. Each molecule has a charge of -17 at physiological pH which contributes to the Gibbs-Donnan effect (see Page 6), greatly increasing the oncotic pressure. In normal humans 5% of intravenous albumin escapes each hour (transcapillary escape) and of this, 10% is metabolised and the remainder returns to the circulation. Two thirds of the exchangeable albumin pool is extravascular, but the majority is held away from the perimicrovascular compartment and therefore does not contribute to the Starling forces. Fifty percent of extravascular albumin is in the skin and accounts for the large protein losses seen in burns.

Solutions of human albumin solution are available for intravenous administration in 4.5% (iso-oncotic) and 20% (hyper-oncotic) concentrations. Theoretically one gram of albumin expands the plasma in normal humans by approximately 18 mL. The hyper-oncotic 20% solution will draw fluid into the plasma from the interstitial compartment because it is so concentrated.

When given intravenously, the concentration of albumin declines with two half lives. The first is of four hours representing transcapillary escape and the second, of 17 days, representing metabolism. The kinetics vary with volume status. Theoretical advantages of albumin as a replacement colloid include binding toxic substances and scavenging free radicals. However, treatment of hypoalbuminaemia with infusions of albumin has not been shown to improve outcome in critically ill patients when compared to synthetic colloids. Furthermore, as solutions of intravenous albumin are expensive, they are not justified for routine volume replacement. Treatment of hypoalbuminaemia with intravenous albumin, although widespread, is now questioned as merely treating the result and not the cause of the pathophysiology. Indeed, serum albumin concentrations correlate poorly with COP and congenital analbuminaemia is quite compatible with life.

There are several potential reasons why infusions of albumin do not improve survival including

- *Adaptation to low concentrations of albumin.* Some humans lack the genes to make albumin. They are almost completely analbuminaemic with a serum concentration of albumin of 1 g/L. These humans appear to survive normally. They do not have any cardiorespiratory dysfunction. The only abnormality is excessive fat deposition in their legs. Studies in analbuminaemic rats suggest that there is a reduced ability to cope with severe environmental stresses compared with normal rats. The mechanism by which these humans adapt to the lack of this important protein is unknown, but increases in other proteins have been reported.

- *Changes in physiology with injury and illness.* It would be surprising if the physiology of critically ill humans was the same as in normals. Indeed, we have shown in critically ill patients that the low serum albumin concentration seen in these patients does not recover in non-survivors, whereas it does in those who survive. In both of these groups albumin was not used to support the circulation, modified gelatin solution being used instead. Colloid oncotic pressure was also measured in both groups of patients. The colloid oncotic pressure was identical in both groups and this may be a reflection of the gelatin molecule from the colloid we gave staying in the circulation. What this study shows is that survivors are able either to reduce the loss of albumin from the circulation or increase its synthesis whereas non-survivors cannot.

- *Changes in the structure of albumin.* Albumin is a highly flexible molecule. It can change shape readily as it picks up ligands and transports them elsewhere in the body. Compounds which bind covalently may alter the structure and function of circulating albumin. Glycosylation of the molecule, such as in diabetes, may alter its uptake into endothelial cells, or across renal glomerular basement membranes. Some parts of the molecule are susceptible to *in vitro* oxidation by free radicals, and subsequent proteolytic hydrolysis. In pancreatitis, enzymatic cleavage of albumin occurs. This also occurs in critical illness. Haemorrhagic pancreatitis releases large amounts of haematin that bind, forming methaemalbumin.

- *Changes in the removal or recirculation of albumin.* Loss of albumin from the circulation is a major reason for its reduction in the early phase of critical illness. It is principally caused by increased leakiness across the endothelial capillary membrane. The precise mediators of this leak are still being discovered and include:

- endotoxin
- cytokines - tumour necrosis factor - alpha (TNF-α and interleukin -6 (1L-6)
- arachidonic acid metabolites C3a and C5a
- complement components
- other vasoactive peptides - bradykinin, histamine
- chemokines - macrophage inflammatory protein 1α (MIP-1α)

With severe illness the pores in the capillaries open allowing albumin to leak into interstitial tissue. The normal transcapillary escape rate can increase by 300% in patients with septic shock, and by 100% after cardiac surgery. Sequestration of the extravascular albumin into non-exchangeable sites may occur, such as into intestinal wall, and into surgical or traumatic wounds. Catabolism of albumin may also be altered. In situations of increased transcapillary albumin flux, an increase in degradation of albumin has been reported. The exact site of catabolism has eluded investigators. It now seems that the vascular endothelium has an important role in albumin degradation.

- *Effects of albumin elsewhere.* There are two major areas where colloids are important. The first is the viscosity of the blood and the second is its clotting (discussed later in this chapter). In laboratory experiments saline mixed with blood produces a lower viscosity compared to starch. Albumin was intermediate.

Albumin has also been investigated in a prospective randomised cross-over study to see if it can cause a diuresis in patients with nephrotic syndrome. Albumin was shown to be of no benefit. Indeed, in subsequent correspondence it was pointed out that the tubular leak of albumin into the capillary may bind to the excreted furosemide, inactivating it. Since furosemide is only active in the free form in the tubule, giving albumin may actually reduce its effectiveness.

Synthetic colloids

Whereas albumin is a colloid with all molecules of equal weight (monodisperse), synthetic colloids (gelatins, dextrans and starches) contain molecules of many different molecular weights (polydisperse). The mean (weight average) molecular weight (MW_w) of these mixtures is the total weight of all molecules divided by the total number of molecules. It tends to be distorted by the larger molecules, some of which may have molecular weights as high as 10,000,000 Da, but which have little oncotic effect. A different measure of these mixtures is the number average molecular weight (MW_n). This is the median of the molecular distribution and indicates the average size of the majority of the oncotically active particles. As the distributions of these preparations are skewed towards lower molecular weight, values of MW_n are smaller than MW_w.

Colloids will have a greater volume expanding effect in a hypovolaemic patient than in a normovolaemic one. In patients with critical illness, the duration of the volume expanding effect is reduced.

Gelatins

Two types of gelatins are available. Succinylated gelatins, (modified fluid gelatins) e.g. Gelofusine® and urea linked gelatins, (polygelines) e.g. Haemaccel®. Their differences are shown in Table 7.

Gelatins are the product of the degradation of animal collagen which is then modified to increase the size of the molecules which improves vascular retention. With succinylated gelatins, NH_3 groups are replaced by charged COO^- groups causing conformational change which increases the size of the molecules. This and the

Colloid	Modified fluid gelatin	Polygelines	0.9% Sodium Chloride
Molecular Weight (Average)	30,000	35,000	58
Concentration	4.0%	3.5%	0.9%
Bonding of gelatin Molecules	Succinylated	Urea linked	N/A
C.O.P. (20,000 Daltons)	40-45 mmHg	25 mmHg	N/A
Negative Charge	34	17	N/A
Calcium (mmol/L)	<0.4	6.25	0
Potassium (mmol/L)	<0.4	5.1	0
Sodium (mmol/L)	154	145	154
Chloride (mmol/L)	120	145	154

Table 7: The differences between modified fluid gelatins, polygelines and 0.9% sodium chloride (N/A = not applicable).

greater negative charge increases the duration of action of modified fluid gelatins compared to polygelines. With urea linked gelatins, smaller molecules are linked to produce molecules of suitable size.

The low calcium content in the modified fluid gelatin makes giving a blood transfusion simpler, immediately after a gelatin transfusion since it is unneccessary to flush the line with saline. With the higher calcium content of polygelines the line must be flushed otherwise the blood may clot. The higher content of potassium in polygelines is also a risk in some patients.

The low molecular weight (MW_w) of 35,000 Da, which is well below the renal threshold can mean a short vascular retention similar to the shorter acting starches. Rapid excretion through the kidneys occurs, where they act as osmotic diuretics. In the patient with renal impairment they may have a greater duration of action. They are of use in situations where short term volume expansion is required, for example to overcome the vasodilatation associated with spinal blockade or the administration of anaesthetic agents. They are also used in the critically ill.

Anaphylaxsis is rare, although it may be marginally higher than the other colloids. Histamine release increases the microvascular endothelial pore size which decreases further the volume expanding effect. Gelatins are presented in 0.9 % sodium chloride, which presents a large sodium load when administered in quantity. In view of the rapid excretion of gelatin molecules, the remaining sodium and water will behave as 0.9% saline and pass into the ECF.

Dextrans

Dextran is a naturally occurring glucose polymer which, unlike other synthetic colloids, is unmodified in manufacture. It is produced from sucrose by *Leuconostoc mesenteroides*. It is available in preparations of MW_w 70,000 Da (Dextran 70) 6% solution and MW_w 40,000 Da (Dextran 40) 10% solution. Both types of solution are available in either 0.9% sodium chloride or 5% glucose. Molecules of dextran are eliminated by the kidneys when the molecular weight is below the renal threshold for dextrans of 55,000 Da. Before administration, 30-40% of dextran 70 and 60-70% of dextran 40 molecules are below this. Larger molecules are broken down by dextranases and are then eliminated by the kidneys. Some uptake of larger molecules can occur in the reticuloendothelial system (RES).

When infused intravenously, dextran 70 has a half life of 6 h. Dextran 40, because of the smaller molecular weight, is rapidly eliminated from the plasma with a half life of 1-2 h. However, being a 10% solution, dextran 40 is hyperoncotic and draws fluid out of the interstitial space, leading to a short plasma expansion. This removal of interstitial fluid is undesirable in dehydrated patients and renal failure may be precipitated.

Dextrans interfere with clotting and have been used in the treatment of post surgical thromboembolic disease, although they are probably less effective than low molecular weight heparin. In the past the use of high molecular weight dextrans was associated with a high incidence of anaphylaxis. This was found to be related to the size of the side chains, which have now been reduced. Dextrans now have a similar incidence of allergic reactions to other colloids.

Starches

A range of colloid products based on hydroxyethyl starch (HES) are available differing on the basis of their molecular weight distribution, substitution and the length of their persistence in the plasma. They are made from amylopectin, derived from corn wax starch, a branched chain glucose polymer. In plasma they are subject to rapid hydrolysis by α–amylase and unmodified would be destroyed within ten minutes. They are also insoluble in water. Addition of hydroxyethyl groups to the glucose subunits increases both solubility in water and resistance to hydrolysis by α-amylase. The degree of substitution is usually expressed as the number of groups per 10 glucose molecules (for example 6 hydroxyethyl groups per 10 glucose molecules is 0.6). The sites available for substitution are 2, 3 and 6 of the glucose molecule (Figure 8). The higher the degree of substitution the more resistant the molecule is to α–amylase.

HES solutions have a very wide range of molecular weights. The concentration of the starch, and its molecular weight determine the extent and duration of action of the solution. A large amount of substitution also enhances this. Substitution into position 2 gives the molecule some resistance to breakdown by α–amylase. However, the greater the degree of substitution the more side effects.

35

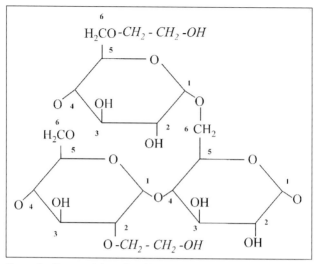

Figure 8: Structural formula of hydroxyethyl starch. $-CH_2 - CH_2 -OH$ is a hydroxyethyl group.

This increased solubility in water is a result of an increased water binding capacity of the molecule which in turn increases its osmotic activity (partially dissolved, semi-hydrophobic molecules do not act as effective solutes as far as osmosis is concerned.). The characteristics of the common starch solutions are described below and summarised in Table 8.

After intravenous administration, individual molecules with a molecular weight below the renal threshold for HES (70,000 Da) will be excreted. Molecules with a molecular weight of greater than this will not initially be excreted, but will be hydrolysed by α-amylase at a rate proportional to the degree of substitution. Products of hydrolysis with molecular weights below the renal threshold will then be excreted.

All molecules, while in the plasma, will contribute to oncotic pressure. Although the larger molecules have very little oncotic activity in their original state, their products of hydrolysis contribute a large number of fresh medium molecular weight molecules. This occurs at a time when the original medium MW molecules have been broken down to below renal threshold size and excreted. This mechanism also contributes to the volume expanding profile of HES. The extent and duration of volume expansion of HES solutions therefore depends on concentration, molecular weight and degree of substitution.

Larger molecules pass into the RES by vacuolation and are metabolised. Many are re-released after breakdown. The extent of RES uptake is difficult to ascertain and accordingly, discrepancies exist in reported figures. This probably reflects a large (15%) but transient initial passage through the RES. Animal studies indicate that very small quantities are present at one week (<3%). This persistence is thought to be of little significance. Passage into the RES is not a major route of elimination of HES.

Starches can be classified according to their molecular weight and substitution. Heta means a substitution of 0.7, while hexa is 0.6 and penta is 0.5. Percentage concentration of the solution is also important. Names of starches often include a description of their substitution. This classification will be used in this text.

Hetastarch
450,000/0.7/6% (Hespan 6% ®)
This has both a high MW_w (450,000 Da) and degree of substitution (0.7) and is therefore characterised by a long persistence in plasma. There is a wide distribution of molecular weights ranging from 10,000 to 10,000,000 Da. The larger molecules are either broken down rapidly by α-amylase in the plasma or more slowly by γ-amylase, which is intracellular. Larger molecules are taken into the RES in the liver and spleen. Vacuolation and transient storage in hepatic parenchymal cells also occur. Hespan has an effect on clotting similar to dextrans.

Pentastarch
200,000/0.5/6% (HAES-steril 6% ®)
This has a medium MW_w (200,000 Da) and DS (0.5). The lower degree of substitution results in a shorter duration of plasma expansion as α-hydrolysis occurs more quickly than with other starches.

200,000/0.5/10% (HAES-steril 10% ®)

This is a hyperoncotic preparation. It is a plasma expander and results in an increase in plasma volume of 130% of the volume infused. This effect is short-lived however and after 3-4 hours the plasma expansion profile is little different from the same starch in a 6% solution.

250,000/0.5/10% (Pentaspan 10% ®)

This has a medium MW_w and a low degree of substitution (0.45) and is presented in a hyperoncotic solution which results in some initial plasma expansion. It has a plasmaprofile similar to HAES-steril but may be eliminated faster.

Hexastarch

2000,000/0.6/6% (EloHAES 6% ®)

This has a medium MW_w (200,000 Da) but has a higher degree of substitution (0.62) than HAES-steril or pentaspan. The importance of the degree of substitution in determining the plasma volume expansion properties of starches during the first 24 hours after administration is illustrated by the similar time course of both hespan and EloHAES. EloHAES has fewer of the very large molecules present in hespan and there will be less prolonged accumulation. It also has less effect on clotting than Hespan.

Pentafraction

This is a special preparation of hydroxyethyl starch which remains under experimental evaluation. All small molecules (<50,000 Da) are removed and the majority of molecules are within a range of 100,000 to 500,000 Da (MW_n 120,000 Da). It should be noted here that with all other colloids (including hespan), the majority of osmotic activity will result from molecules that are smaller than this. The purpose of this particular distribution is that the majority of molecules will be retained within the plasma even when injury has given rise to increased microvascular permeability. It has also been postulated that plugging of leaky capillaries may occur.

Concentration(g/L)		MW$_w$	MW$_n$	DS	COP (mmHg)
Hespan 6%®	60	450	70	0.7	27
HAES-steril 6%®	60	200	70	0.5	34
HAES-steril 10%®	100	200	70	0.5	80
EloHAES 6%®	60	200	60	0.62	25-30
Pentaspan 10%®	100	264	63	0.45	55-60
Gelofusine®	40	30	22.6	-	40-45
Haemaccel®	35	35	15	-	25
Dextran-40	100	40	25	-	160
Dextran-70	60	70	39	-	78

Table 8: Properties of colloid solutions. MW$_w$ is the weight average molecular Weight, MW$_n$ is the number average molecular weight, DS = degree of substitution and COP is the colloid osmotic pressure.

Coagulation and volume expansion

Both crystalloids and colloids have effects on coagulation. All of the reports of these effects have been related to surgery or *in-vitro* tests. This may not be applicable to all patients, especially those critically ill, for the following reasons.

- There may be a coagulopathy caused by the disease which is exacerbated by the crystalloid/colloid.
- Elimination of the colloids may be abnormal in the critically ill because of renal and hepatic dysfunction.
- The pore size in the vascular endothelium may be abnormal and this will result in an alteration of the duration of effect

Gelatins may change blood coagulation by several mechanisms. They appear to interfere with fibrin polymerisation resulting in a weak clot of reduced mass. They also act by inhibiting platelet aggregation. It should also be noted that both albumin and fibrinogen also do this.

The effects of gelatins and starches on coagulation have been compared. During cardiopulmonary bypass there was no difference in effect on clotting between a 200,000/0.5 starch and gelatin. However, there was a significant difference between a 450,000/0.7

starch and gelatin. The HMW starch caused a reduction in platelet aggregation.

The effect of extreme haemodilution during surgery using HAS has been studied. Little significant effect on platelets and fibrinogen was seen but a combined deficiency of other factors was measured. Some authors have suggested that albumin is the "golden standard" inferring that it has little or no effect on coagulation. However, based on clinical observations albumin has been shown to have a heparin-like effect and to reduce platelet stickiness

In other studies HAS has been compared to starches and gelatins. In patients given HAS an increase in von Willebrand factor was seen compared to a normal level seen in the others.

Starches also affect blood coagulation in several ways. First, like all fluids used for resuscitation they may dilute the clotting factors in the blood. Second, there may be interference with the release of von Willebrand factor and factor VIII. Starches may also accelerate the conversion of fibrinogen to fibrin. Accelerated clot formation may result in a weak clot.

The increase in pore size which occurs during critical illness increases the renal threshold from 60,000 Da to approximately 100,000 Da. This will result in a marked reduction in the oncotic activity of albumin in these patients, perhaps explaining why it is no better than gelatins in these patients. The MW_n of starches is also below 100kDa although these preparations contain some activity above this. Pentafraction (experimental) was designed with a MW_n of c. 200,000 to overcome this.

The clinical importance of these effects on coagulation remains to be elucidated.

Making sense of the crystalloid/colloid debate

Which fluid to use when resuscitating patients is a controversy that has raged for over 20 years and it is still going! There are two main groups, those who use large volumes of crystalloids and those who use smaller volumes of colloids.

Intravenous resuscitation became widespread during the second world war. In the years following the war it was realised that salt and water were retained after trauma and surgery and it became customary to restrict them. Blood alone was given to replace blood loss. This resulted in seriously hypovolaemic patients as other causes of perioperative plasma volume loss were not appreciated, for example; insensible and evaporative losses, tissue sequestration, accumulation of fluid in the bowel and movement of fluid into "sick cells."

In the 1960's Shires showed that patients who received crystalloids and blood did better than those who received blood alone. In an attempt to explain this finding, he showed a contraction of the interstitial compartment during haemorrhage using radioactive tracers in a laboratory study of bleeding in animals. This was then also shown to occur in trauma and during major surgery. As crystalloids are distributed throughout the ECF, their value was attributed to the resuscitation of this contracted compartment (Figure 9). Shires' findings that the functional interstitial space is contracted have been disputed by others. It is obviously difficult to apply the steady state measurements of tracer distribution Shires used to what is clearly a very unstable situation.

Three possible mechanisms have been proposed to explain the contraction of the interstitial compartment.

- After moderate haemorrhage, a shift of fluid into the plasma occurs from the interstitial compartment (plasma volume refill) at a rate of 90 to 120 mL/h. This is partly a result of altered Starlings forces (low P_{mv}) and is also a result of a sympathoadrenally mediated increase in pre- and post-capillary resistance ratio.
- Increases in intracellular osmolarity, secondary to cell hypoxia, resulting in movement of fluid and electrolyte from the extra cellular compartment to the intracellular compartment causing intracellular overhydration.
- Movement of fluid away from the parenchymal subcomparment into *non-exchangeable subcompartments* within the interstitial compartment (third space) is thought to occur. It remains here as oedema, but it's extracellular physiological function is lost.

Given this situation Shires thought that it would be logical to use crystalloids to resuscitate both the intravascular and interstitial compartments. The initial controversy that this caused in the 1960's was in fact with those who believed that water and electrolytes were retained during the perioperative period with an expansion of the interstitial compartment and should therefore be restricted. Retention of water and electrolytes undoubtedly occurs in relation to stress mediated hormonal changes associated with surgery and anaesthesia. However, plasma volume deficits in these patients are greater than was then realised and the benefits of restoring plasma volume and maintaining delivery of oxygen and nutrients to the tissue with large volumes of crystalloid were overwhelming. Fluid restriction is now no longer an issue in perioperative patients.

> Hypovolaemia causes renal failure.
> This is more difficult to treat than fluid overload

A major concern with the administration of large volumes of crystalloids is that it will lead to pulmonary oedema. In a healthy lung this will only occur when very large amounts are given which exceed perimicrovascular lymphatic drainage which is extremely efficient in the lung. In addition, administration of crystalloids will lead to parallel changes in both Πmv and Πpmv (Page 8 - Starling - Landis equation) and therefore crystalloids are more likely to

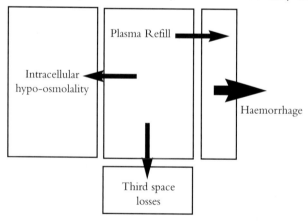

Figure 9: Schematic diagram of the possible fluxes of fluid away from the ECF during acute haemorrhage - as proposed by the proponents of crystalloid resuscitation of this space.

remain in the vascular compartment after haemorrhage. Consideration of the Starting Landis equation shows that alterations in hydrostatic pressure ΔP are then of greater importance than changes in oncotic pressure $\Delta \Pi$ in determining fluid flux across the pulmonary microvascular endothelium.

Administration of crystalloids in critical illness and adult respiratory distress syndrome (ARDS) is more problematic and is considered further in Chapters 5 & 6.

The controversy which followed in the 1970's related to whether deficits in plasma volume were better treated with colloids which were believed to expand better that compartment. Some of these arguments are summarised in Figure 10.

For Crystalloids

Cheap – even with large volumes
No anaphylaxsis
Resuscitate the interstitial space

For Colloids

Smaller volumes needed
  • Faster to give
  • Less thermal stress
  • Less sodium load

Figure 10: The balance of arguments for and against crystalloids and colloids.

Colloids certainly now have an important place in plasma volume expansion although their use varies widely internationally depending on the prevailing practice. The main argument for the use of colloids is that they rapidly result in plasma expansion with a return of haemodynamics and tissue perfusion, hopefully preventing release of organ injury mediators which result in increases in microvascular permeability. It is important to appreciate, however, that not all colloids are equally effective in this regard. The use of large volumes of gelatins, for example, to replace blood loss on a volume for volume basis may result in late hypovolaemia as the volume expanding effect has a half life of only 2-3h.

> The speed of effective resuscitation is far more important than the type of fluid used.
> In a shocked patient use what is available rather than searching for a specific fluid.

The question of the contracted interstitial space remains unresolved, it is regarded as vitally important in the United States where balanced electrolyte solutions (page 26) (and blood when necessary) are used in quantity for resuscitation in trauma, haemorrhage and perioperatively with the explicit aim of restoring the interstitial compartment. Many authorities subscribing to the colloid school of thought regard this as unimportant and therefore view crystalloid regimens as irrational.

If the interstitial space becomes depleted it is likely to do so in previously healthy individuals during the acute insults of haemorrhagic shock or trauma/major surgery. Even if colloids are preferred for rapid plasma volume expansion, one must still ask if the interstitial space needs resuscitation. In later stages, as fluids are given and as water and electrolytes are retained, extravascular fluid and electrolyte depletion is less likely to be a problem.

The crystalloid/colloid controversy remains important as practice varies widely throughout the world depending upon which view is taken. A balanced appraisal is difficult as most of the available research and reviews on this subject fall strongly into one camp or the other. Both types of fluid when used appropriately are, however, highly effective.

Which colloid when?

Unfortunately there is no simple answer to this question. Much of the evidence about colloids is either old or conflicting. Although several recent meta-analyses have given apparently clear indications about what to use and more importantly what not to use (see for example *British Medical Journal* 1998 317:235) they are based on flawed evidence. This does not mean they should be ignored. We have used the best evidence available, interpreting the results with caution. Unfortunately, this means that the choice of fluid is dictated by personal experience, and sometimes by cost. We are as guilty of this as others and our recommendations need to be interpreted in the light of local policy.

- We rarely use albumin. There is evidence that its use does not improve survival, pulmonary oedema, renal failure, or any other measure of outcome in adults. Serum concentrations of albumin appear to be an indicator of the underlying disease state. Giving albumin to increase these concentrations does not treat the underlying disease. In the future groups may be identified for whom it is of value. At the moment we only use it in patients who have an acute fulminant liver injury and after abdominal paracentesis for ascites. Animal work suggests that liver cells may recover less slowly if gelatins are used. Used after paracentesis the changes in the renin/angiotensin system are less.

- Gelatins are the mainstay of our volume resuscitation policy. They appear to offer the best compromise between efficacy, safety and cost.
- We use starches in certain patients, however their use is limited by the maximum volume that can be prescribed in each 24h. Occasionally they can produce pruritus that can be long lasting and distressing for the patient.
- We have stopped using dextrans. They can cause difficulty with cross-matching, anaphylaxsis (but no more frequently than gelatins) and are no more effective than other solutions.

Shock

A single definition of shock that satisfactorily describes all the different types is difficult. One of the best definitions is shock is a state in which there is an insufficient delivery of oxygen to the cells. Needless to say cellular hypoxia is difficult to diagnose at the bedside! Instead, changes in heart rate and blood pressure are amongst the common early warning signs along with oliguria, cold peripheries and sometimes mental confusion. These and other common signs of shock are summarised in Table 9.

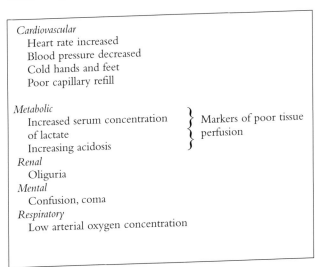

Cardiovascular
    Heart rate increased
    Blood pressure decreased
    Cold hands and feet
    Poor capillary refill

Metabolic
    Increased serum concentration   } Markers of poor tissue
    of lactate   } perfusion
    Increasing acidosis   }
Renal
    Oliguria
Mental
    Confusion, coma
Respiratory
    Low arterial oxygen concentration

Table 9: Common signs of shock.

Heart rate and blood pressure (BP) are the signs which most commonly change and one usually affects the other.

Blood pressure
This depends upon the cardiac output and the systemic vascular resistance (SVR). If the cardiac output goes down blood pressure can be maintained by increasing the systemic vascular resistance (vaso-constriction). This explains the cold hands and feet seen in shock. Conversely, if the systemic vascular resistance goes down because of vasodilation (for example in septic shock) then the hands and feel will feel warm.

Blood pressure $\propto$ cardiac output $\times$ systemic vascular resistance.

Cardiac output
The cardiac output (CO) is the product of heart rate (HR) $\times$ stroke volume (SV). The stroke volume is the amount of blood ejected by the heart with each beat (Figure 11)

Heart rate
Usually the faster the heart beat the greater the cardiac output. However, at very high heart rates (>120-160/min) the time during diastole may be so short that the heart cannot fill properly and cardiac output goes down.

Stroke volume
The volume of blood ejected with each heart beat will depend upon:

- Preload
  The more a heart muscle fibre is stretched the greater will be the force of contraction. Heart muscles can be stretched by increasing the amount of blood in the chambers. This increase in volume results in an increase in pressure. Since the amount of stretching of a muscle fibre cannot be measured the increase in pressure of the blood is used instead. Two pressures are commonly used - central venous pressure (CVP) and pulmonary artery occlusion pressure (PAOP). These are described later under monitoring.

- Inotropy
  This describes the strength of the heart muscle. It may be weakened by ischaemia, toxins etc. When the inotropic activity of the heart is decreased stroke volume decreases.

- Rhythm
  To pump efficiently, the atria need to have their systole during ventricular diastole. This allows the ventricles to have the maximum preload before ventricular systole starts. Any arrhythmia that stops the coordination between the atria and the ventricles will reduce cardiac output.

Afterload
If the SVR decreases then the work of the heart is reduced. This in turn allows an increase in stroke volume. Conversely, if the SVR increases then stroke volume will decrease.

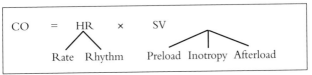

Figure 11: Factors affecting cardiac output.

Oxygen delivery

The definition of shock at the beginning of the chapter gives importance to the delivery of oxygen to the cells. At the moment there is no easy way to measure this. Whole body oxygen delivery (DO_2) is the best we can measure. Oxygen delivery (DO_2) depends on the cardiac output, haemoglobin (Hb) and oxygen saturation. (SaO_2). (The 1.84 is the volume of oxygen (mL) that binds to 1 g of haemoglobin.) Instead of measuring Hb, SaO_2 and assuming the amount dissolved is a function of these many arterial blood gas machines now measure oxygen content directly.

$$DO_2 = CO \times \text{Oxygen content of the blood (Hb} \times SaO_2 \times 1.84)$$

At one time oxygen delivery was increased to "supranormal" levels using catecholamines. This practice is now decreasing. However, the concept of an adequate cardiac output, sufficient haemoglobin and avoidance of hypoxaemia remains a cornerstone of good resuscitation.

Resuscitation

There is no single treatment for shock. However, nearly all types of shock (with the exception of cardiogenic shock) usually need some degree of expansion of the circulating blood volume. This may be because of the loss of fluid from this compartment (such as bleeding) or because the compartment has got bigger (such as is seen with the vasodilation of sepsis). Whatever the cause the principles of volume resuscitation are the same. One of the most important principles is that when considering cardiovascular variables, isolated values are of less importance than trends.

> Use trends rather than isolated readings of cardiovascular variables.

Before treatment can be explained monitoring needs to be understood.

Monitoring

Arterial pressure

The pressure required for adequate renal perfusion is usually about 100 mmHg systolic. In younger patients the threshold figure may be lower; in previously hypertensive patients it may be much higher.

> Try to find out the patient's normal blood pressure

It is often possible to review the blood pressure and urine output chart and note which arterial pressures have been associated with good hourly urine volumes. The lowest of these figures can be set as a target for future therapy.

Peripheral circulation

As blood is lost so the blood supply to non-essential organs is reduced. The decrease in cardiac output causes adrenergic stimulation reducing blood supply to the skin as well as other organs. The vasoconstriction leads to cold and clammy peripheries. This can be measured by recording the rectal (core) and toe (peripheral) temperature. The difference between the core and periphery may reach 2°C.

Urine output

Patients should make 1 mL/kg/h of urine. The management of oliguria is described in Chapter 7.

Central venous pressure

The assumption that the pressure in the great veins and the right atrium is related to blood volume (Page 48) may be justified at values of less than 5 cm H_2O. For example, a patient with a CVP of 2 cm H_2O is likely to be hypovolaemic. However, as an isolated measure, CVP is too unreliable as there are many other factors affecting the result.

CVP is best used in conjunction with a fluid challenge. (Figure 13). Alternatively, it can be measured with the patient lying and then remeasured with them sitting. A decrease of 5 cm H_2O suggests hypovolaemia.

> It is possible to have a CVP > 5 cmH$_2$O and still be hypovolaemic.

CVP measurement must be made with care to avoid levelling errors and false increases from infusions of drugs, fluids etc. into the same line. CVP recording may be poorly done on a general ward, and hourly urine volumes will be a much more reliable guide to fluid therapy for most patients. In the oliguric, postoperative patient, without cardiac failure, the CVP should be maintained at a minimum of 10 mmHg (13 cmH$_2$O). This is a useful threshold whether the patient's lungs are mechanically ventilated or breathing spontaneously.

Pulmonary artery catheter monitoring

The pulmonary artery catheter (PAC) is a fine tube with several lumens. These lumens may be used for measuring pressures in various parts of the heart, such as the pulmonary artery and right atrium. A lumen is also used to inflate/deflate the balloon at the tip. Other lumen may contain a small electrical wire to a thermistor, also at the tip of the catheter used to measure the temperature of the blood.

The PAC is inserted through a large vein in the neck or the groin. The balloon is blown up and the catheter floated through the veins, right atrium and right ventricle until it is in the pulmonary artery. Here the catheter is further advanced until the balloon wedges in the pulmonary artery. Characteristic waveforms (Figure 12) allow the location of the catheter to be recognised.

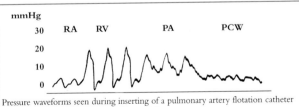

Pressure waveforms seen during inserting of a pulmonary artery flotation catheter
RA = Right atrium, RV = Right ventricle
PA = Pulmonary artery, PCW = Pulmonary capilliary wedge

Figure 12: The pulmonary artery catheter. Characteristic wave forms.

Once correctly placed the balloon is deflated. Several measurements can be made. These include:

- Pulmonary artery occlusion pressure (PAOP).
  Inflating the balloon occludes blood flow from the right side of the heart. When the balloon is inflated the distal (end) lumen in the pulmonary artery is connected to the left ventricle through the pulmonary artery, arterioles, capillaries, venules, vein and left atrium. This enables the filling pressures of the *left side* to be measured.

  Errors are easily made if the zeroing and the waveforms are not carefully checked. For any circulatory change, changes in PAOP are greater than for CVP. It is therefore a more sensitive monitor of therapy. Use of PAOP also eliminates errors arising from pathology in the right heart and pulmonary circulation.

Digital displays of physiological variables are too easy to believe and sometimes wrong.

Waveforms must <u>always</u> be checked and zeros established before acting on any CVP or PAOP observation.

A target of PAOP between 12-15 mmHg will normally assure an adequate circulating blood volume.

- Cardiac output measurement
  The thermistor at the tip allows cardiac output to be measured. With the balloon deflated a cold solution of 5% glucose is injected into the right atrium. As the bolus of cold blood containing the glucose passes the thermistor the reduction of temperature is measured along with its duration. A computer calculates the cardiac output from this.

  Cardiac output can be divided by the body surface area to give cardiac index (CI). This should be the same for all adults irrespective of size.

  Measurement of cardiac index allows estimation of the systemic vascular resistance index (SVRI), which may be low in the septic patient. If the patient is hypotensive with an adequate cardiac index (greater that 2.4 L/min/m²) the SVRI will be low.

Treatment with low doses of α-adrenergic agonists e.g. norepinephrine (0.03 μg/kg/h) may restore renal perfusion and urine output where fluid replacement has been confirmed as adequate by CVP or PAOP measurement.

General guidelines for the management of shock.

Shock is a serious condition that causes significant morbidity and mortality. Expert help should be sought early on if:

- Simple measures do not rapidly improve the patient.
- The patient is desperately ill when first seen.

> No good ICU doctor minds an invitation to review a patient who rapidly improves with simple care, so not needing admission to the ICU.
>
> All ICU doctors dislike being called when shock has been present, but inadequately treated, for a long time and as a consequence the patient will have a prolonged stay in the ICU with multiple organ failure.

The following are steps that should be taken in shocked patients:
If the patient is unconscious, breathing inadequately or cyanosed.
- Support the patient's breathing using a self-inflating bag
    — Intubate the trachea
    — *If you do not know what to do call an anaesthetist or ICU doctor*
- Give oxygen 6 litres/min by face mask
- Make sure you have good intravenous access
- Find out the likely cause for the shock, if it is not cardiogenic shock then the patient is probably hypovolaemic
- Give fluid (0.9% saline, gelatin, starch etc) until a response is seen unless the patient has cardiogenic shock. The use of an automated blood pressure machine can be invaluable in obtaining frequent recordings to allow reassessment.
- A central venous catheter may be useful to guide resuscitation and avoid over- or under-filling. Aim for a CVP of at least 10 mmHg (13 cmH$_2$O).
- Review your treatment frequently. Aims are shown in Table 10.
- Insert a urinary catheter, empty the bladder and then measure hourly urine output.

Heart rate less than 100
Systolic blood pressure +/- 15% of normal (or at least
> 110mmHg)
Urine output > 1mL/kg/h
Haematocrit > 30%.

Table 10: Indicators of adequate resuscitation.

In some patients it may be unclear if they are still hypovolaemic or not. The flow chart in Figure 13 may help.

Types of shock
There are several different causes of shock that all doctors may encounter. These are:

Haemorrhagic shock
Because this is so common and involves relatively complicated fluids (blood and its components) it has been given its own chapter (Chapter 6).

Cardiogenic shock
Cardiogenic shock is a result of an impairment of the pump function of the heart. This may occur after a myocardial infarct or during severe myocarditis. Plasma volume is usually unchanged. Failure to pump blood results in an increased hydrostatic pressure in the lungs (raised PAOP) and great vessels (raised CVP). Fluid therapy in this situation may be harmful. Indeed, further volume may reduce the cardiac output and/or cause pulmonary oedema.

Treatment of the circulatory disturbance includes the use of:
- Inotropic agents such as epinephrine, dobutamine.
- Vasodilators to lower the SVR so increasing cardiac output. In addition these will also increase the intravascular space reducing the effective blood volume.
- Diuretics to excrete excess salt and water.
- Treatment of arrhythmias to improve the heart's pumping action.
- General measures for myocardial infarction, such as aspirin.

Septic shock and systemic inflammatory response syndrome (SIRS)
Septic shock is a result of vasodilation secondary to the release of inflammatory mediators (endotoxin, TNF II-6 etc.). It is mediated by nitric oxide in the microvascular membrane. In more severe

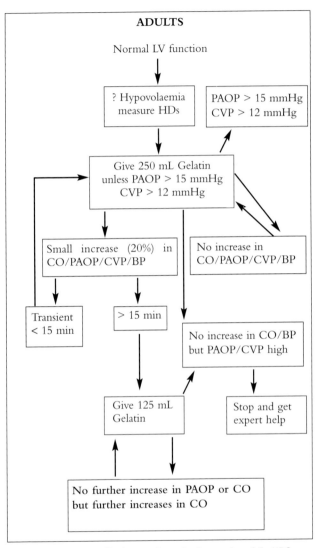

Figure 13: Unsure if the patient is hypovolaemic? HDS = Haemodynamic measurement. Cardiac output is best, then wedge pressure, then CVP followed by blood pressure.

cases, there will be impairment of pump function superimposed (cardiogenic shock). The cardiovascular management of septic shock requires a careful balance of vasoconstriction and fluid resuscitation, guided by frequent (invasive) assessments of cardiovascular function. Systemic inflammatory response syndrome (SIRS) produces a clinically indistinguishable impairment of circulatory function. In addition to the classical signs of shock described at the beginning of this chapter disturbances in liver function, blood clotting etc. may be seen. As well as volume resuscitation the following points need remembering:

- Investigate the sepsis. Blood cultures, body fluids, wounds, swabs etc. should be sent to the microbiology laboratory.
- Treat the sepsis. Start antibiotics, drain any pus.
- Hypovolaemia is common because of vasodilation and because the capillaries become "leaky" allowing fluid to escape from the circulation (Page 8).
- Myocardial depression may occur caused by the release of toxins. This may need inotropic drugs (as for cardiogenic shock above).
- Acute adrenal failure may occur needing physiological doses of steroid (25 mg hydrocortisone 6 hourly).

Anaphylactic shock
Anaphylactic shock is the result of a sudden massive increase in capillary leakiness with a shift of fluid to the ECF and a loss of plasma volume. In addition, massive vasodilatation will occur.

This is caused by a foreign protein or drug being given which results in an acute and inappropriate release of inflammatory mediators. The response can be rapid and life threatening. Some of the signs and symptoms are shown in Table 11.

The immediate treatment is to give epinephrine. 0.5 mg IM repeated if neccessary 5 minutes later if there is no improvement. Usually there is a large fluid loss into the skin and other tissues as well as profound vasodilation. Large amounts of fluid may be needed.

Other treatments include:
- Give hydrocortisone (100 mg) and antihistamines (chlorpheniramine 10 mg) to reduce the effects of the anaphylaxsis, although the value of these is unproven.

Cardiovascular
  Tachycardia
  Hypotension
  Cardiac arrest

Respiratory
  Bronchoconstriction
  Angioneurotic oedema

Skin
  Hypoxaemia
          Cyanosis
          Mottling
  Local Histamine release
          Erythema
          Wheals

Table 11: Some of the symptoms and signs of anaphylaxis.

- Early tracheal intubation orally or by tracheostomy if there is laryngeal swelling.
- Administration of β agonists for wheeze.
- Early tracheal intubation for severe wheeze not responding to β agonists.

Once the patient is stable blood is taken for various investigations including a tryptase. This is a measure of mast cell degranulation which always occurs in anaphylaxsis.

Neurogenic (spinal) shock
Neurogenic (spinal) shock is a result of the vasodilatation which follows the loss of sympathetic tone following a high spinal cord lesion. A similar picture may be seen with high spinal (epidural/subarachnoid) anaesthesia. Both fluid and vasoconstrictors may be required.

Histotoxic shock
Histotoxic shock is a result of a specific poisoning of respiratory enzyme systems, for example by cyanide. It requires specific treatment and is not a fluid balance problem.

Bleeding

Bleeding is a common emergency in medical practice. Early treatment is essential, delay risks death, which even if not immediate may follow as a consequence of multiple organ failure. Expert help is usually needed to assess the need for urgent operation; this chapter contains the basic information for "first aid". Amongst the commonest reasons are trauma, surgery (including post-operative bleeding) and bleeding from the gastro-intestinal tract such as from varices or an ulcer. The effect this will have on the patient will depend upon the condition of the patient (the older or sicker the patient the greater the effect) and the amount of blood lost.

The response to blood loss

Every text book dealing with this subject describes the classical physical signs associated with blood loss. However, often these are confused by other conditions such as pain or pre-existing disease. This should be remembered when reading the description below.

Heart rate
An increase in heart rate is often the first sign of acute blood loss. This response attempts to maintain cardiac output. Fortunately, it is also the easiest to measure. However, it is also affected by many other things, for example pain from a fracture.

Signs of peripheral vasoconstriction
This is shown by the patient having cold peripheries (hands and feet) with peripheral cyanosis and a slow capillary return. There is a mottled appearance on the skin.

> Tachycardia and signs of peripheral vasoconstriction are the earliest signs of haemorrhagic shock.

Respiratory rate
Respiratory rate is a sensitive sign in bleeding patients. It will be increased to 20-30 in a patient who has lost 1000 mL. It may be >30 in a patient who has lost 2000 mL.

Blood pressure
This does not change when the blood loss is small. As loss increases to >750 mL the diastolic pressure will increase, narrowing the pulse pressure This is a result of sympathetically mediated vasoconstriction. Systolic pressure is maintained until the blood loss exceeds 1500 mL in most patients after which it decreases. In fit young adults peripheral vasoconstriction may occur and even in the presence of severe blood loss blood pressure may be maintained (or even slightly increased). When this occurs there is always a tachycardia. Other signs will also be present.

> The rule of 100:
> If the heart rate is over 100 and the blood pressure below 100 the patient is hypovolaemic.

Although this simple rule can be wrong on occasions, if applied intelligently it is an invaluable guide.

It is important to try and relate the blood pressure of a patient losing blood to their normal blood pressure. Particularly in the elderly a blood pressure of 110/70 mmHg may represent profound hypotension because the patient is normally hypertensive.

> Try to find out the patient's normal blood pressure and base treatment on that.

Urine output
When fluid is lost from the body and the circulating blood volume is reduced the body tries to conserve water by excreting a low volume of urine with a high concentration of solutes. There are several mechanisms for this, in particular a marked increase in the

excretion of renin, angiotensin and antiduretic hormone (Page 107).The latter leads to an increase in urinary specific gravity. Hourly urine volume is a useful guide to adequacy of resuscitation. The minimum is 0.5 mL/kg/h, but it is better to aim for 1 mL/kg/h.

Haemoglobin and haematocrit
The measurement of haemoglobin or haematocrit to estimate blood loss is unreliable and should not be used for this purpose. During acute blood loss it may take up to three days for the compensatory haemodilution to occur. If blood is being transfused then it will reflect the blood being given rather than acting as a guide to the amount of blood being lost.

Although haematocrit and haemoglobin do not help in telling how much fluid or blood to give, they may help guide which fluid to give during resuscitation. If the haematocrit is less than 30% or the haemoglobin less than 10 g/dL then blood is needed.

Patients who are bleeding are constantly changing and need frequent reassessment. Ongoing treatment must be guided by the patient's reponse to initial therapy.

Some of the physiological changes associated with bleeding are shown in Table 12. For the estimates for blood loss an assumption that a 70 kg man has about 5 L of blood (70 mL/kg) has been made.

Further information about resuscitation can be found Chapter 5.

Site of blood loss
Often it is obvious where blood is being lost from. On occasions a source of bleeding may not be obvious. If so, examine the patient carefully paying particular attention to the following:

- *Chest*. Large amounts of bleeding can occur into the chest, usually from trauma. This may follow obvious trauma, such as a road traffic accident, with a fractured rib causing bleeding from an intercostal vessel for example. However, bear in mind that several "medical" procedures may also produce "silent bleeding" into the chest. This includes chest drain insertion, aspiration of a pleural effusion and central venous line insertion.
- *Abdomen*. Bleeding may occur from anywhere in the gastrointestinal tract including oesophageal varices, ulcers, arterio-venous

malformations, tumours etc.

- *Fractures.* Torrential bleeding, without an external source, may occur from a fractured pelvis. Bleeding from bilateral fractured femurs can also be potentially life-threatening, 1.5 - 2 litres being lost in each leg.

---

1   15% (0.75 L)
    No measurable changes in BP, pulse pressure or respiration.
    Variable HR and signs of poor peripheral perfusion.

II 15-30% (0.75 - 1.5 L)
    Tachycardia >100   Tachypnoea 20-30
    Decreased pulse pressure.
    Anxiety.

III 30-40% (1.5 - 2 L)
    Marked tachycardia >120   Tachypnoea 30-40
    Fall in systolic blood pressure.
    Marked mental changes with confusion.
    Oliguria.

IV > 40% (>2 L)
    Tachycardia >120
    Marked fall in systolic pressure, often with an unrecordable diastolic pressure.
    Confused with impaired consciousness.
    Anuria.

Table 12. Summary of changes of blood loss. (Adapted from Advanced Trauma Life Support Student Manual, 1993, 5th Edition, American College of Surgeons, Chicago.)

What to use

There are three choices. Crystalloids, colloids or blood. The debate about crystalloids and colloids is discussed elsewhere (Page 40). However, when faced with a profoundly shocked patient give whatever is available rather than debate or have to find a "special" solution.

- Do not use glucose solutions as volume expanders. They are mostly water and are very inefficient.
- (0.9% sodium chloride or balanced electrolyte solutions (Page 26) (Hartmann's) are effective crystalloids for use on the resuscitation of hypovolaemia.

Blood should be given to maintain a haematocrit of about 30%. This will ensure that there is sufficient oxygen carrying capacity in the blood to keep the tissues healthy. Bear in mind that giving blood is not without risk. It is a biological product and this carries several risks including:

- Protein incompatibilities from:
  - — An incompatible blood transfusion.
  - — White blood cells - reactions may be caused by sensitisation to human leucocyte antigens, usually the result of previous transfusion or pregnancy.
  - — Donor plasma proteins - this is rare and may result in febrile or non febrile reaction with out haemolysis. They can be life threatening.
- Infection, bacterial and also with viruses such as hepatitis B, C, (non A, non B), cytomegalovirus, HIV and rarely Epstein- Barr virus.
- Hypothermia - because blood contains living cells it needs to be refrigerated to prevent deterioration.

The Blood Bank

The first person to transfuse blood from one human being to another was Dr J Blundell in 1829 who transfused 227 mL of blood into a patient who had had a serious post-partum haemorrhage. The first modern blood bank was established in 1937 at the Cook County Hospital, Chicago, by Bernard Fantes. The functions of today's blood bank include:

- Obtaining, testing, typing, labeling, storage, cross-matching and issuing blood.
- The preparation of blood products such as platelets, fresh frozen plasma, cryoprecipitate.
- The long-term storage of blood cells and blood products, such as frozen blood.
- In conjunction with the haematology laboratory tests of coagulation to enable the proper selection of blood products.

Blood component therapy

Blood may be stored as whole blood which has a haematocrit of 40%. Alternatively, plasma, platelets and other components may be removed. When plasma is removed the concentrated red cells remaining will have a haematocrit of 60%. It is this that is usually given out by the blood bank when blood is requested. The normal storage time for blood is 28 days.

Platelet concentrates
These are prepared by differential centrifugation either from freshly drawn units of blood or from donors who give larger quantities of platelets by plateletphoresis. The storage time of platelets is relatively short, about 6-7 days. The indication for platelets is usually bleeding. Occasionally they may be given prophylactically. If the patient is bleeding then they should be given when the platelet count is $<80,000 \times 10^9$/L. A similar value is usually required before surgery.

Fresh frozen plasma
This is also obtained when the unit of blood is donated. It is immediately deep frozen to protect its factor V and VII. Its indications are
- Massive blood transfusion.
- Urgent reversal of the effect of warfarin.
- Replacement of isolated factor deficiencies when the laboratory evidence supports this.

Cryoprecipitate
This product contains high levels of fibrinogen and factor VIII. It is mostly used in the treatment of patients with haemophilia. It can however be used occasionally for patients with massive blood transfusion if the fibrinogen level is <1 g/dL.

Blood storage
When blood is stored several precautions have to be taken:
- The blood should be tested to be as free as possible from infection.
- It needs to be clearly labelled for type etc.
- It should not clot.

To prolong its shelf life, (by reducing energy demands) it needs to be kept at between 1-6°C.

Several methods can be used to stop clotting. One of the commonest is acid citrate dextrose (ACD). The citrate binds calcium, inhibiting coagulation. Dextrose is a substrate for the red blood cells, maintaining glycolysis. The acid acts as a buffer to stop the pH

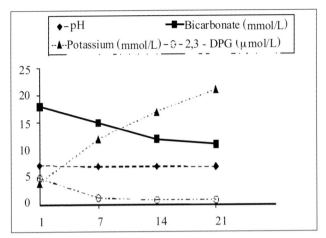

Figure 14: Changes in the plasma of stored blood. Redrawn from Stoelting RK and Miller RD. Fluid and Blood Therapy in: *Basics of Anaesthesia* 3rd. edn. Chapter 17. Churchill Livingstone. New York 1994.

decreasing too much during storage. As storage continues so changes in the plasma occur. These are shown in Figure 14.

Adenine has been added to CPD (CPDA) to prolong storage. Other storage solutions contain adenine, glucose, mannitol and sodium chloride (Adsol®) or glucose, adenine, citrate, phosphate and sodium chloride (Nitricel®). For really long-term storage blood can be deep frozen.

Effects of storage on coagulation
Clotting factors
Nearly all of these are stable except factors V and VIII. These decrease by 85% and 50% respectively by 21 days. Platelet count is usually only 10% of normal after 24 h and quickly decreases to zero after that.

Compatibility testing
Blood is typed as being AB, A, B or O and rhesus positive or negative. Giving the wrong blood–group blood to the patient can have fatal consequences because of antibodies to the AB, A, B, O proteins. The same type of blood as that of the patient's should not

Donor	Recipient
O	O, A, B, AB
A	A, AB
B	B, AB
AB	AB

Table 13: Compatibility of different blood groups.

produce a reaction. However, other blood types may be compatible with the patient. Table 13 shows compatibility between blood groups.

Patients who are rhesus positive can receive rhesus positive and negative blood, whilst those patients who are rhesus negative can normally only receive rhesus negative blood.

In addition to screening for blood types and rhesus compatibility blood also needs to be screened for unusual antibodies such as Kell, Kidd and Duffy. The usual way to ensure that a unit of banked blood is compatible with the patient is to take a small sample of the recipient's serum and mix it with a selection of red cells. If they are incompatible then agglutination will occur.

Three types of blood transfusion are possible.

1. Immediate transfusion of blood needed to save a patient's life because of severe haemorrhage. O–negative blood should be given while other blood is being cross–matched. Until cross–matched blood is available only O negative blood can be given.

2. Group compatible. In this instance the patient's blood group and rhesus state are known. Compatible blood is obtained from the blood bank. Note however, that historical information (for example in the notes) is occasionally wrong and therefore the group is always checked by the laboratory before the blood is issued. This takes about 5 minutes.

3. Full cross-match. This takes about 20 minutes. Blood groups, major and minor incompatibilities will have been excluded.

The risk of blood transfusion decreases from 1 to 3. Unnecessary use of 1 and 2 hazards the patient by increasing the risk of a mis-matched transfusion.

More recent methods of blood transfusion have dramatically reduced the times for cross matching blood using automated processes. For example both donor and recipient blood may be typed for ABO group and screened for antibodies so long as this does not show any incompatibility or abnormality then cross-matching may be omitted (type and screen).

Transfusion reactions

These are rare. Some are unavoidable, unfortunately most are the results of a mistake. Over half of all the mistakes involve doctors or nurses doing something wrong after the blood has been issued from the blood bank. Death occurs in about 1 in 100,000 transfusions and haemolytic reactions in 1 in 4-6,000. These can occur with as little as 10 mL of blood.

Fever is the commonest sign. It may be associated with chills, chest pain, hypotension, flushing nausea, haemoglobinuria and the development of a bleeding tendency.

---

1. STOP THE TRANSFUSION
2. Maintain the urine output at a minimum of 75 to 100 mL/h by the following:
   a. Give fluids intravenously to ensure the patient is not hypovolaemic.
   b. Mannitol, 20 g given over a 15 minute period.
   c. If a and b are ineffective, give furosemide, 20 to 40 mg, intravenously.
3. Prevent hypotension to ensure adequate renal blood flow.
4. Alkalinize the urine; since bicarbonate is preferentially excreted in the urine, only 1 mmol/kg of sodium bicarbonate is usually needed to increase the urine pH to 8. After 30 min repeat the urine pH to see if more bicarbonate is needed.
5. Measure platelet count, partial thromboplastin time, and serum fibrinogen level
6. Return unused blood to blood bank for re-crossmatch.
7. Send a repeat blood sample to the blood bank for an antibody screen and direct antiglobulin test.

Table 14: Steps for the treatment of the renal complications of a haemolytic transfusion reaction.

Renal failure may follow as a consequence of haemoglobin deposition in the renal tubules. A suggested regimen for dealing with this problem is shown in Table 14.

Hazards of massive blood transfusion

Although infusing large amounts of blood into patients who are bleeding is life-saving, it is not without risk. Some of the hazards include

Decrease in body temperature

- Blood is stored at 4°C. This will cool the patient unless it is warmed first.
- In addition, the patient will lose heat to their environment because of exposure, for example after a road traffic accident, or because their abdomen or chest is open in the operating theatre.

The effects of a reduction in body temperature are many. These include:

- A decrease in cardiac output, which may worsen the shock.
- The clotting factors are enzymes. These work less well when the patient is cold. This will exacerbate bleeding.
- The liver makes less clotting factors when it is cold.
- In the same way platelets do not work well when the patient is cold. Again this will exacerbate bleeding.

To prevent the patient from getting cold in the emergency department they should be covered with a clear polythene sheet or a space blanket. In the operating theatre warming blankets or hot air blowers should be used. The same method should be used after operations. At all times warmed fluids should be given.

Dilutional coagulopathy.

- Stored blood is low in factors V and VIII. This needs to be replaced by the use of fresh frozen plasma (FFP). If there are no laboratory results for guidance we recommend giving two units of fresh frozen plasma for each 10 units of whole blood. In many parts of the world blood banks no longer issue whole blood. Instead, concentrated red cells may be issued. Then more fresh frozen plasma may need to be given. The exact amount of FFP depends on:

- The rate of blood loss and transfusion. Rapid transfusion (> 4 units of red cell concentrate/h) will probably need the rate quoted here, rates of transfusion of blood less than this may need smaller amounts of FFP.
- The temperature of the patient. If the patient is cold then the liver will be less able to make clotting factors.
- Platelets do not last for more than 24 hours after collection of blood. Thrombocytopenia may develop as a consequence. Platelets should be given based on laboratory results. However, as many patients are taking aspirin for the prevention of myocardial infarction and cerebrovascular insufficiency its effects on platelet function needs to be remembered. Aspirin will reduce platelet "stickiness" for up to 14 days. Absolute values of platelet count may be unreliable.
- Acidosis. The anticoagulant used in blood by many blood banks is acid citrate dextrose (ACD). Not surprisingly infusion of blood containing this anticoagulant leads to an acidosis in the patient. In addition, poor tissue perfusion, if there is shock, causes many tissues in the body to function anaerobically. This produces more acid, especially lactic acid. Finally, because the liver and kidney are also underperfused they are unable to eliminate any build up of acid. Routine administration of sodium bicarbonate is not recommended. If the base deficit is >10 mmol/L, the patient is shocked and unstable, small (50 mmol) aliquots over 10 min may be useful. Usually the acidosis corrects itself as the bleeding stops, when resuscitation is complete and the tissues are adequately perfused.
- Potassium - as blood is stored so potassium leaks out of the cells. The longer the blood is stored for, the greater the potassium concentration. This is rarely a problem in patients with normal renal function. However, the use of blood that has been stored for a long time infused into patients with poor renal function may result in hyperkalemia.
- Hypocalcaemia - the citrate in ACD may bind calcium. This will reduce its ionized or free fraction. This can result in a reduction of cardiac output. It may also result in arrhythmias. Note that most laboratories measure total calcium concentration which includes that which is bound to citrate as well as albumin. Ionized calcium should be measured. If it cannot be measured then watch the T waves on the ECG. If they become peaked the patient may be hypocalcaemic; give the patient 10 mL of 13.4% calcium chloride.

- Micro aggregates. As blood is stored so debris, platelets and red blood cells may form small clumps. These may not be removed by the 170 μM filter in a giving set. If these particles are infused into the patient then they will be filtered out in the pulmonary circulation. Here they may cause an inflammatory reaction resulting in the acute respiratory distress syndrome (ARDS). This may cause hypoxaemia necessitating high oxygen concentrations and mechanical ventilation. It may be exacerbated by the underlying injury the patient suffered. The risk of this can be reduced by using a blood filter that only allows particles of about 40μM to go through it. Bigger particles are collected in the filter. More recently buffy coat depleted blood has become available, that does not need filtration or leucocyte.

What to do when faced with a patient with a massive haemorrhage

The first thing to do is not to panic! A little blood spilt over a bed, on the floor or the road goes a long way. Remember the basics - airway, breathing and then circulation. However, shock is a medical emergency which should be treated as such. If you are out of your depth, cannot get intravenous access, do your best but send for help early. The following are some guidelines:

- Put in one, preferably two, 14 gauge intravenous catheters. Good sites for these are the antecubital fossae. If the patient has major trauma consider a third intravenous catheter in the leg in case there has been damage to the great vessels from the arms. If these are damaged then any blood you infuse may not get into the circulation, leaking out where the vessel is damaged. Small gauge cannulae (e.g.< 18 G) should not be used. They have too much resistance to flow. Poisseulle's law states that for each doubling of the radius flow will increase 16 times.
- As you put in one of these intravenous cannulae take off blood for base line laboratory investigations and cross-matching.
- If the patient is severely shocked in the first 1-2 minutes infuse whatever fluid is nearest to hand and give it quickly.
- After the infusion of 2 litres of fluid reassess the situation and decide which fluid to continue.
- Give the patient 4 litres of oxygen by face mask to ensure there is sufficient oxygen getting to the blood.

- Cover the patient with a polythene sheet to prevent heat loss.
- At the earliest opportunity warm all fluids. This means putting a blood warmer up into the circuit. A blood warmer simply warms fluid as it passes through hot water or between metal plates. Some fluids may be kept in a warm cupboard.

> Do not microwave blood, blood products, gelatins, starches or dextrans. Doing so may degrade them and make them toxic.

What to aim for during resuscitation

Guidelines for suitable end points to aim for during bleeding are shown in Table 15.

> Heart rate less than 100.
> Systolic blood pressure +/- 15% of normal
>   (or at least > 110 mmHg).
> Urine output > 1 ml/kg/h.
> Haematocrit > 30%.

Table 15: Some indicators of adequate resuscitation.

Perioperative blood transfusion

It used to be thought that all patients with a haemoglobin level below 10 g/dL having a general anaesthetic needed a blood transfusion first. This view has now been challenged and the minimum acceptable haemoglobin concentration before operation is now recognised to depend on several factors. These include:

- *Type of operation.* If the planned operation does not have a risk of heavy blood loss then a lower starting haemoglobin is acceptable.
- *Age of patient.* Younger patients tolerate a lower haemoglobin level better than the elderly.
- *Presence of ischaemic heart disease.* To compensate for a lower haemoglobin and a reduced oxygen carrying capacity the cardiac output must increase to maintain oxgen delivery. Patients with ischaemic heart disease may not be able to tolerate this increased work load. Angina or myocardial infarction may result.

- Pre-existing disease. Some diseases, such as chronic renal failure, may enable the patient to tolerate a lower than normal haemoglobin. Others, such as ischaemic heart disease (see above) may limit the degree of anaemia tolerated.

In a patient who is deemed in need of correction of the anaemia before surgery, the operation should be postponed if possible and the anaemia corrected medically. If the surgery is urgent or is to treat a condition which is causing the anaemia, perioperative blood transfusion may be required. It is of note that up to 70% of all blood transfusions are given in the perioperative period.

It is easy to cross match blood, even when it is not needed. This leads to wastage and inefficient use of blood. To reduce this the Maximum Surgical Blood Ordering Schedule (MSBOS) was introduced at Addenbrooke's Hospital.

The schedule lists the number of units of blood routinely issued for elective surgical procedures. It is based on retrospective analysis of usage associated with these procedures. It aims to correlate the amount of blood issued or crossmatched (C) to the amount of blood transfused (T). The C:T ratio can be used to monitor the efficiency of the scheme. The ideal value for the C:T ratio is 1.0, but a more realistic objective is 2:1. This corresponds to a blood usage of 50%.

The schedule is shown below (by kind permission of Mr Brian Tolliday, Principal MLSO, Addenbrooke's Hospital).

Surgical procedures normally fall into two categories:
1. Group and antibody screen only (G&S)
2. Units issued according to the schedule

The system allows flexibility. If patients in the G&S category have a positive antibody screen, antigen negative blood must be cross-matched. If the clinical circumstances indicate that extra blood may be needed, the schedule can be exceeded. However, exceeding the schedule is monitored to prevent abuse of the system.

Maximum surgical blood ordering schedule
Group and save procedures

ENT/ORAL
Cleft lip repair
Cleft palate repair
Tonsillectomy

**GYNAECOLOGY
OBSTETRICS**
Antepartum haemorrhage
Abortion
Abruption
Caesarean section
Colposuspension
Cone biopsy
Dilation and curettage
Oophrectomy
Pelvic floor repair
Reversal of sterilisation
Sterilisation
Total abdominal
    endometrial resection
Tubal surgery
Vaginal repair
Ectopic pregnancy
Salpingectomy
Trial of labour/scar
Postpartum haemorrhage
Placenta praevia
    (type 1 & 2)

ORTHOPAEDICS
Above knee amputation
Below knee amputation
Pugh nail
Removal of femoral nail

UROLOGY
Cystoscopy
Neck of bladder incision
Nephrolithotomy
Renal biopsy
Ureter reimplantation
Ureteric implant
Urethroplasty

NEUROSURGERY
Discectomy
Cranioplasty
Cloward's procedure
Cervical
    decompression
Fossa exploration
Lobotomy
Neuroma removal
Parotidectomy
Shunt revision
Spinal fusion
Thyroidectomy
VA shunt
VP shunt
Blocked shunt
Burr hole biopsy
LamInectomy

**THORACIC/
CARDIAC**
Angioplasty

GENERAL
Angiography
Bowel resection
Breast reduction
Breast excision
Cholangiogram
Cholecystectomy
Closure of colostomy
Colostomy
Embolectomy
Endoscopy
ERCP
Grafting of burns
Haemorroidectomy
Hemicolectomy
Hiatus hernia repair
Highly selective
    vagotomy
Ileostomy

Liver biopsy
Laparoscopy

Laparotomy
Mastectomy
Myelogram
Pyleoplasty
Polyps removal
Rectopexy
Sclerotherapy
Splenectomy ★
Tracheostomy
Varicose vein
    removal

★ unless large
spleen

Maximum surgical blood ordering schedule: how much blood to cross match

ENT/ORAL SURGERY

Pharyngoplasty	2
Laryngectomy	2

GYNAECOLOGY/OBSTETRICS

Radical vulectomy	3
Wertheims Hysterectomy	4
Placenta praevia (type 3 & 4)	4
Ruptured ectopic pregnancy	2

ORTHOPAEDICS

Thompson's prosthesis	2
Knee replacement	2
Total hip replacement	3
Bilateral hip replacement	4
Revision of THR	6
Harrington's rod	3
Fractured neck of femur	2
Osteotomy	2

THORACIC/CARDIAC

Aortic aneurysm repair	6
Aorto-iliac disobliteration	10
Pulmonary lobectomy	2
Cardiac artery bypass graft	6
Left/right valve replacement	6
Mitral/atrial valve replacement	6
Fem/popliteal bypass	2

UROLOGY

Nephroureterectomy	4
Uretherolithotomy	2
Transurethral resection of prostate	2
Transurethral resection of bladder tumour	2
Nephrectomy	2
Cystectomy	4

NEUROSURGERY

Craniotomy	2
Meningioma excision	6
Aneurysm clipping	4
Lobectomy	2
Acoustic neuroma removal	4

GENERAL

Abdo perineal resection	2
Anterior resection	2
Gastrectomy	2
Park's pouch	2
Portacaval shunt	4
Hemihepatectomy	10
Liver transplant	20
Renal transplant	2
Pancreas transplant	10
Bone marrow harvest	2
Whipple's operation	4
Oesophagectomy	4
Colectomy	2
Colonic resection	2
Sigmoid colectomy	2
Panproctocolectomy	2
Hartman's procedure	2
Splenectomy	2★

★ if spleen is large

Blood transfusion after operation

Postoperatively, similar constraints apply. A further change is occurring with one unit transfusions. In the past this was frowned upon, since one unit transfusions were thought to be of no value. Now, clinicians are starting to realise that if there is a "target" haemoglobin and the patient falls below it why give two units of blood when one would suffice? Giving two just because they are available doubles the risk. However, more important is to decide if the target haemoglobin needs rethinking! Giving no blood gets rid of the risk of transfusion altogether!

Oliguria

Oliguria is defined as an hourly urine output of less than 0.5 mL/kg/h for two consecutive hours, or a urine output of less than 400 mL in 24 h. The importance of oliguria is that it is a warning sign. Ignored, renal failure may occur. In the majority of cases oliguria can be treated simply by the administration of fluid. However, in too many cases the situation is exacerbated by the administration of nephrotoxic drugs to "at risk" patients. The aim of treatment is to prevent renal failure by preserving and rapidly restoring renal blood flow.

The maximum concentrating power of the kidney is 1200 mosmol/kg and a minimum of 500 mL urine in 24 h is therefore required to excrete the obligatory daily solute load of 600 mosmol. Whilst oliguria may represent the physiological response to dehydration, it may also be a sign of impending renal failure. Prompt investigation and treatment are necessary to prevent renal damage and the onset of established renal failure.

> The prevention and prompt correction of oliguria is easier than the treatment of renal failure.

This chapter does not describe the treatment of renal failure nor the management of fluid and electrolyte balance in this situation. Readers of this book should not attempt this, but obtain expert help.

Causes of oliguria

The causes of oliguria may be classified in the same way as renal failure which is divided into three groups, prerenal, renal and postrenal. In patients several factors may act together (Figure 15).

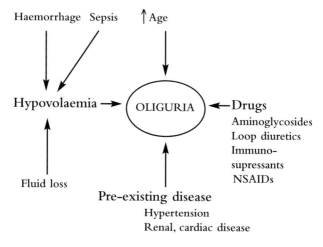

Figure 15: Some of the common factors that may predispose to oliguria in patients.

The causes of pre-oliguria are shown in Table 16.

Prerenal

Renal hypoperfusion causes a reduction in glomerular filtration rate without parenchymal damage. Increased reabsorption of sodium and water leads to the production of a concentrated urine with a low urinary sodium. It is usually reversible by fluid replacement, which restores renal blood flow if treatment is started promptly.

> More patients suffer because of too little fluid than from fluid overload.

Renal

Acute renal failure is caused by an intrinsic renal cause in about 30 - 40 % of cases. In the majority of these cases it is because of prolonged renal hypoperfusion or nephrotoxins. The risk is increased when hypotension is associated with sepsis. In contrast to prerenal oliguria, there is damage to the tubular epithelium, a condition known as acute tubular necrosis. The initial event in acute tubular necrosis is a 50% reduction in renal blood flow leading to a reduction in glomerular filtration rate and tubular ischaemia.

Damage to the renal vascular endothelium disrupts the physiological balance between endothelin induced vasoconstriction and nitric oxide induced vasodilatation. The resulting vasoconstriction persists after the initial insult has passed and is not immediately reversible by fluid resuscitation. In addition to vasoconstriction, excessive endothelin activity encourages adhesion of the leukocytes to the endothelial cells causing congestion of the capillary and impeding flow along it.

The thick ascending limb of the Loop of Henle in the renal medulla is most prone to damage in acute tubular necrosis, because the oxygen tension in the medulla is normally low and the cells have a high oxygen requirement for active transport of solute. Ischaemic damage causes cellular necrosis which results in obstruction of the tubular lumen by casts and cellular debris. This allows a back leak of filtrate from the tubular lumen into the interstitium. Following the development of acute tubular necrosis there is an oliguric or anuric phase that lasts from two to six weeks followed by recovery of renal function and the production of large volumes of dilute urine.

NSAIDs

Oliguria and renal failure following the use of non steroidal anti-inflammatory drugs (NSAIDs) is well recognised. Prostaglandins, especially prostaglandin PGE_2 and PGI_2 are produced in the kidney. Under normal physiological conditions they have little effect on renal function. Their release is stimulated by hypovolaemia, when concentrations of norepinephrine or angiotensin II are high to maintain renal blood flow and glomerular filtration rate. NSAIDs inhibit the synthesis of prostaglandins and the kidney is vulnerable to ischaemic damage when renal blood flow is reduced.

PRE RENAL OLIGURIA

Low cardiac output:
Cardiogenic shock, myocardial infarction, congestive
cardiac failure, cardiac tamponade, pulmonary embolus, arrhythmias
Peripheral vasodilation:
Anaphylaxis, drugs, sepsis
Excess fluid loss from:
Gastrointestinal tract:vomiting, diarrhoea, ileus, intestinal obstruction,
peritonitis
Kidneys: diuretics, diabetes insipidus, osmotic diuresis
Skin: burns, sweating
Haemorrhage: Concealed or obvious, trauma, post surgery
Vascular occlusion:
Renal artery stenosis, embolus,
thrombosis, aortic dissection, vasculitis

INTRINSIC RENAL CAUSES OF OLIGURIA

Glomerular:
Membranoproliferative glomerulonephritis
Secondary glomerulonephritis: systemic lupus
erythrematosus, Goodpasture's syndrome, Wegener's
granulomatosis
Acute interstitial nephritis:
Allergic: Methicillin, NSAIDs, sulphonamides, captopril, furosemide,
rifampicin, trimethoprim
Radiation
Acute tubular necrosis: Ischaemia (see prerenal failure)
Toxins: aminoglycoside antibiotics, radiographic contrast agents,
amphoteracin, paracetamol, cyclosporine, FK506, heavy metals, organic
solvents, fluoride, ethylene glycol
Intratubular pigments: Free haemoglobin, myoglobin
Intratubular crystals: Uric acid

POST RENAL CAUSES

Ureteric:
Papillary necrosis, calculi, tumour, blood clot
Abdominal or pelvic tumour
Retroperitoneal fibrosis
Accidental ureteric ligation
Abdominal tamponade: blood, ascites, surgical packs
Bladder:
Tumour
Neurogenic bladder
Blood clot
Prostatic hypertrophy
Urethra:
Stenosis, stricture, trauma

Table 16: Causes of oliguria.

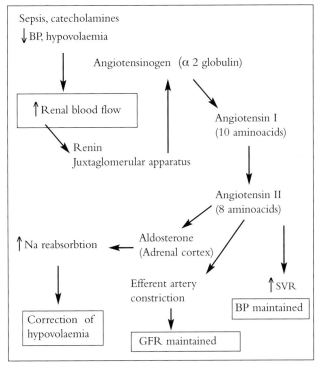

Figure 16: The effects of hypoperfusion of the kidney.

Aminoglycosides
The aminoglycoside antibiotics are nephrotoxic. The risk is dose related and is greatest in the elderly and patients with renal failure. Therapy should be guided by regular measurement of plasma concentrations in patients with impaired renal function.

ACE inhibitors
Although they are not directly nephrotoxic, angiotensin converting enzyme inhibitors (ACE inhibitors) should not be used in patients with known renovascular disease. In patients with bilateral renal artery stenosis ACE inhibitors markedly reduce glomerular filtration and cause renal failure.

Intrinsic causes
The intrinsic causes of acute renal failure are shown in Table 16.

Postrenal

This implies obstruction in the ureters, bladder or urethra. Postrenal causes account for less than 10% of cases of renal failure, but should be excluded as a cause of oliguria because most causes are treatable. They are shown in Table 16.

Management

It is easier to prevent oliguria than to treat established renal failure and it is therefore important to recognise at risk patients. The combination of hypotension and hypovolaemia predispose to oliguria. This risk is increased in the presence of sepsis, especially if the patient has been hypotensive for a prolonged period of time. Patients undergoing emergency surgery are often dehydrated and adequate fluid resuscitation before surgery is essential to prevent oliguria.

Aminoglycoside antibiotics and NSAIDs should be used with caution in elderly patients who are more susceptible to the effects of hypovolaemia.

Avoid the combination of
- Hypotension
- Non steroidal anti-inflammatory drugs
- Gentamicin

Especially in the elderly orthopaedic patient
Monitor aminoglycoside levels

In patients with impaired renal function, the serum creatinine only increases above normal values after the glomerular filtration has decreased by 40-50%. These patients therefore have little renal reserve. Patients with chronic hypertension are at increased risk from hypotension as the renal blood flow autoregulation curve is shifted to the right.

Find out the patient's normal blood pressure. Use this to base treatment on rather than what you think is normal.

The principles of the management of oliguria (Table 17) are to treat any life threatening complications, establish the cause, correct hypovolaemia (see Chapter 6) and restore renal blood flow in order to promote a diuresis.

Treat any life threatening consequences (hyperkalaemia)
Establish the cause
Stop all nephrotoxic drugs (aminoglycoside antibiotics, ACE inhibitors, NSAIDs)
Exclude urinary tract obstruction (check catheter, bladder washout, renal ultrasound)
Assess state of circulation and hydration
Fluid challenge
Restore circulating blood volume and normal blood pressure
Initiate diuresis (diuretic, mannitol, dopamine)
Maintain diuresis (urine output of 1 mL/kg/h)

Table 17: The management of oliguria.

Diagnosis

History

A history should be obtained from the patient, noting any symptoms of chronic renal disease such as polyuria, fatigue or hypertension. Recent drug treatment together with a fever, rash and arthralgia are suggestive of interstitial nephritis. The case notes should be examined for previous blood pressure recordings and electrolyte or urinalysis results. Anaesthetic and fluid balance charts should be reviewed noting daily input and output and the cumulative fluid balance. These are often inaccurate and may underestimate fluid loss, as insensible losses, fluid sequestered in an ileus or as oedema will also not be recorded. Drug charts should be scrutinised for nephrotoxic drugs.

When reviewing a patient with renal impairment always look at the fluid balance and drug chart

Examination

The patient should be examined to assess their state of hydration and the adequacy of the circulation. Tachycardia is a good sign of hypovolaemia, but pain or anxiety may sometimes make the interpretation difficult. Blood pressure usually decreases with increasing hypovolaemia. However in young people compensatory mechanisms will try to maintain the blood pressure until hypovolaemia is extreme leading to rapid circulatory collapse. Skin turgor, sunken eyes and dry mucous membranes are subjective signs and poor indicators of hydration.

The adequacy of the circulation should be assessed. Simple clinical examination should be performed before more invasive monitoring is used. The blood pressure should be recorded and compared to the patient's normal blood pressure An impaired level of consciousness may indicate a low cardiac output. The peripheral perfusion should be assessed by noting the temperature and perfusion of the hands and feet. Cold peripheries in the clinical setting of hypovolaemia means that the circulation is inadequate and that the patient is attempting to maintain their blood pressure by vasoconstriction. The abdomen should be examined to exclude abdominal tamponade caused by blood, ascites or intestinal obstruction.

If the patient's condition does not respond to simple treatment measures, or there are other organ systems that need support, the patient should be referred to a high dependency or intensive care unit for invasive monitoring of central venous pressure (CVP), arterial pressure and pulmonary capillary wedge pressure (Chapter 5).

Investigations

Blood should be taken for urea and electrolytes, serum creatinine and serum osmolality. A urine sample should be taken for microscopy, culture and osmolality.

Urinalysis may be a guide in differentiating between a prerenal and a renal cause of oliguria (Table 18). The urinary sodium is low if there is a prerenal cause as the body tries to retain sodium in order to maintain the circulating blood volume. A high urinary sodium is found in acute tubular necrosis or glomerular disease. Recent administration of furosemide or mannitol which decrease reabsorption of sodium in ascending limb of the loop of Henle will make the interpretation of urinary electrolytes difficult. Treatment should not be based on the biochemical results alone, but take into account the clinical situation.

	Prerenal	Renal
Urine osmolality (mosmol/kg)	>500	<350
Urine/plasma creatinine ratio	>40	<20
Urine/plasma urea	>8	<4
Urinary sodium (mmol/L)	<20	>40

Table 18: Differences in the urinary biochemistry in prerenal and renal oliguria.

Microscopic examination of the urine sediment may show hyaline casts if the cause is prerenal. In acute tubular necrosis there are cellular and tubular casts. Pigmented casts are found in rhabdomyolysis. Red blood cell casts are found in glomerular disease or vasculitis and eosinophils in allergic interstitial nephritis.

A markedly increased serum creatine phosphokinase should alert the clinician to a diagnosis of rhabdomyolysis and the urine should be tested for the presence of myoglobin.

A renal ultrasound should be performed to exclude obstruction of the upper urinary tract and to determine the size of the kidneys. Small kidneys may indicate long standing renal disease.

If the abdomen is distended, intra-abdominal pressure may be measured using a urinary catheter. The bladder is emptied and 50 mL of 0.9% saline is put into the bladder. A water manometer as used for measuring central venous pressure is connected to the catheter via a three way tap. Intravesical pressure which correlates with intra-abdominal pressure can be measured using the symphysis pubis as a reference point. The value of the measurement is discussed on Page 90.

Active Treatment

> Treat oliguria early, do not wait until the patient is anuric

Any life threatening complications of oliguria such as severe hyperkalaemia greater than 6 mmol/L must be treated immediately. Although laboratory measurement of the serum concentration is the most reliable in some circumstances the changes of hyperkalaemia can be seen on the ECG may be of value (Table 19). It is important to realise these act only as a guide and may be missing with profound hyperkalaemia.

Serum K$^+$ mmol/L	ECG change
6	Tall peaked T waves
6-8	Widening of QRS complex. Prolongation of the PR interval, loss of P wave
> 8	S wave merges into T wave, sine wave pattern leading to cardiac arrest

Table 19: Signs of hyperkalaemia on the ECG.

The treatment of hyperkalaemia is shown in Table 20.

Treatment	Onset	Duration
Calcium chloride 10% 10 mL iv over 1 min	1 min	1 h
Soluble insulin 10 units + 50% glucose 50 mL iv over 20 min	15-30 min	3 h
Sodium bicarbonate 8.4% 50-100 mL iv over 15 min	30 min	1-2 h
Cation exchange resins Resonium A, (Calcium Resonium) 15 g 6 hrly orally or 30 g rectally	240 min	12 h

Table 20: Management of hyperkalaemia

If not already in place, a urinary catheter should be inserted and an hourly measurement of urine output together with accurate fluid balance chart should be started. An obstructive cause of oliguria must be excluded. The sudden onset of anuria with a catheter in place suggests a blocked catheter and the position and patency of the catheter should always be checked. It is surprising how often oliguria can be cured by a bladder washout! Obstruction of the upper urinary tract may require drainage by percutaneous nephrostomy. The intra-abdominal pressure should be measured if the abdomen is distended and surgical decompression should be considered if the pressure is greater than 30 cm H_2O.

No urine output

- No catheter
- Catheter in the wrong place
- Catheter blocked
- Surgical trauma e.g. ligation of ureters
- Renal vascular pathology (e.g. aortic dissection, renal artery embolus)
- Ruptured bladder

Fluid challenges in Oliguria

The commonest cause of oliguria is hypovolaemia. Assessing the adequacy of fluid resuscitation is difficult. There are no absolute values that must be reached and therapy should be tailored to the individual patient's response. A fluid challenge is used to assess the intravascular volume. An infusion of 250 mL of fluid over 15 min. is used and the response is noted, see Page 55. Colloids such as Gelofusine® or Haemaccel® which remain in the intravascular compartment longer than crystalloids are more efficient and smaller volumes are required, see Chapter 4. All measures of circulating blood volume, blood pressure, pulse rate, peripheral perfusion and urine output should be used to assess the effect of the challenge. The aim of treatment is to resuscitate the patient to their normal blood pressure with no tachycardia and warm peripheries (Chapter 5).

If there is no response to two fluid challenges a central venous catheter should be inserted. An absolute figure for the CVP is less important than the change in value after the challenge. However care should be taken when performing a fluid challenge in a patient with an elevated CVP (>12 cm H_2O, 16 mmHg).

The commonest cause of an "elevated" CVP when it is measured using a water manometer is a blocked catheter, or a zero point that is too high or too low.

Smaller volumes of fluid should be used in patients with known cardiac or pulmonary disease. These patients should be considered for referral to an intensive care unit for insertion of a pulmonary artery catheter to guide fluid replacement.

An attempt to initiate a diuresis should only be made after the patient has been resuscitated with fluid (Chapter 5) or any existing hypovolaemia will be worsened. A summary of drug doses is found in Table 21.

Small bolus doses of furosemide 10-20 mg iv are often very effective. Starting with a large dose may promote an excessive diuresis and lead to hypovolaemia. If there is no response to a small dose of furosemide, a bolus of 80 mg may be given. Larger doses may be required in patients taking diuretics regularly. High doses of furosemide (250 - 500 mg) must be given at a rate of no more than 4 mg/min as they can cause deafness and cardiac arrest. An infusion of 5-10 mg/h of furosemide may increase urine output, but should only be used in a high dependency or intensive care unit. There is no evidence however that the use of an infusion of furosemide prevents the onset or shortens the duration of renal failure.

Mannitol is an osmotic diuretic that often promotes a diuresis. It is useful if there has been severe tissue damage or a reperfusion injury.

Although still widely used, there is no evidence that infusions of "renal dose" dopamine (2-5 μg/kg/min) prevent renal failure. Dopamine has two main effects on the kidney. It is an inotrope and increases cardiac output and renal blood flow due to β_1-receptor stimulation. This action may occur at low doses. It also acts on the renal tubules and promotes sodium excretion causing a natriuresis and diuresis. Like other inotropes, its use may be harmful in patients who have not been adequately volume resuscitated. Current evidence shows dopamine should not be used as prophylaxis to prevent renal failure, but it may increase urine output and maintain a diuresis, which will make fluid management easier. A diuresis does not always mean that the glomerular filtration rate has increased. However, if the patient has sustained tubular damage and is not able to concentrate their urine, the diuresis will increase solute excretion. Large volumes (80-100 mL/h) may be needed to maintain solute balance in patients with impaired renal function.

Drug	Dose	Comments
Furosemide	10-250 mg iv	Start with low doses (10-20 mg), give doses >250 mg at 4 mg/min
Mannitol 20%	0.25 g/kg iv	Give over 15 min, caution in fluid overload
Dopamine	2 µg/kg/min	200 mg in 50 mL 5% glucose

Table 21: Drugs used in the treatment of oliguria.

If the urine output does not increase with the treatment discussed above, the fluid input should be reduced to match the urine output and the electrolytes monitored regularly to detect hyperkalaemia. The patient must be referred as soon as possible to a renal, or intensive care physician for further management.

Rhabdomyolysis
Rhabdomyolysis is increasingly recognised as a cause of oliguria (Table 22). Acute destruction of skeletal muscle leads to the liberation of myoglobin. Myoglobin precipitates in the renal tubules causing acute tubular necrosis.

Exercise, trauma, crush or compartment syndrome, tourniquets, hypothermia, malignant hyperthermia, burns, electric shock, status epilepticus, polymyositis, viral infections, snake and spider venom, ethanol, amphetamines, cocaine, LSD

Table 22: Causes of rhabdomyolysis.

Rapid treatment of rhabdomyolysis is crucial to prevent renal failure. Early treatment may protect the kidney. Our regimen is shown in Table 23.

Start treatment as soon as possible
Prompt resuscitation and restoration of circulating blood volume
Mannitol 20% 0.25 g/kg, if passing urine
Maintain urine output >100 mL/h
Keep urine pH alkaline (>pH 7) NaHCO$_3$ 25 mmol/h
Treat for 3 days or until myoglobin disappears from urine

Table 23: Management of rhabdomyolysis.

THEORY

Physiology

The renal blood flow is 1.2-1.3 L/min which is 25% of the cardiac output. This is maintained by autoregulation and hence glomerular filtration is constant over a wide range of systemic arterial blood pressures. However, if the mean arterial pressure falls below 60 mmHg renal blood flow and glomerular filtration rate decreases rapidly. Renal perfusion is determined by the mean arterial pressure minus the renal venous pressure.

The renal perfusion pressure can be reduced by a decrease in systemic blood pressure, as in shock, or an increase in renal venous pressure. The latter may occur if, for example, the intra-abdominal pressure increases above 20 cm H_2O leading to a decrease in renal perfusion pressure and oliguria.

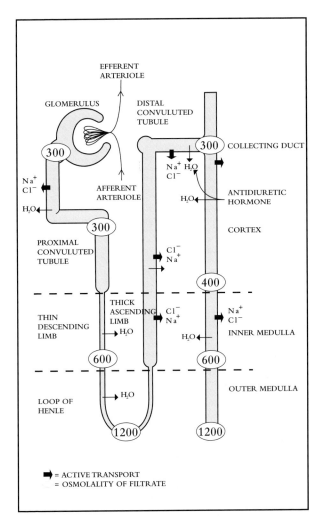

Figure 17: The kidney.

Maintenance of an adequate circulating blood volume and a normal blood pressure is therefore essential to maintain renal perfusion and prevent the development of renal failure. About 90%

of the renal blood supply goes to the cortex. Only 10% goes to the medulla in order to maintain the osmotic gradients and increase urine concentration. Even in the normal kidney the blood supply to the outer medulla is barely sufficient to meet demand. The cells of the medulla are therefore particularly vulnerable to a reduction in renal blood flow.

The kidneys of a normal adult filter about 180 L/day which gives a glomerular filtration rate of 125 mL/min. As the normal urine output is about one litre per day, 99% of the filtrate is reabsorbed. Sixty to seventy per cent of the filtered sodium and water is reabsorbed in the proximal convoluted tubule. Sodium reabsorption is an active process and the reabsorption of chloride and water are passive and linked to the active transport of sodium.

The descending limb of the Loop of Henle is permeable to water. Water passes out of the tubule into the hypertonic medullary interstitium and the tubular fluid becomes hypertonic. In the thick ascending limb of the Loop of Henle a further 25% of the filtered sodium reabsorbed. This process is energy dependent occurring through the action of the sodium potassium ATPase. The enzyme is inhibited by the action of furosemide. Because the ascending limb is relatively impermeable to water, more sodium than water is absorbed and a hypotonic tubular fluid is produced.

The distal convoluted tubule, which is relatively impermeable to water, has a similar function to the thick ascending limb of the Loop of Henle and removes solute in excess of solvent. In the cortical section of the collecting ducts antidiuretic hormone, secreted by the posterior pituitary gland in response to changes in serum osmolality, increases the permeability of the collecting ducts to water. Thus when antidiuretic hormone is secreted more water is reabsorbed and less excreted in the urine. Further water is removed in the medullary collecting ducts as the filtrate passes through the hypertonic medullary interstitium. In this way a concentrated urine with a maximum osmolality of 1200 mosmol/L is produced.

Patients before and after surgery

Patients having surgery are one of the commonest groups needing intravenous fluids. Management of patients before emergency surgery often necessitates resuscitation. Afterwards fluid administration must provide for the basic maintenance requirement together with the anticipated losses in the postoperative period. Then continuing observation will determine any further needs.

Preparing the emergency patient for surgery
Anaesthesia and surgery are very safe today. However, the risk of both is significantly increased if patients are hypovolaemic before surgery. This is commonly caused by:

- Bleeding
- Vomiting and diarrhoea, especially when combined with an inability to drink or absorb fluids.
- Losses into obstructed bowel.
- Sepsis.

Bleeding is dealt with in Chapter 6. However in some instances the need for life-saving surgery will take precedence over full resuscitation.

In some instances of torrential bleeding immediate surgery takes precedence over resuscitation

---

The remaining causes commonly involve an intra-abdominal emergency. In this case there is usually time to resuscitate the patient adequately before the operation. It is essential to do this, failure to do so results in an increased morbidity and mortality.

In patients with an acute abdomen, resuscitation before operation reduces morbidity and mortality

---

The morbidity and mortality may not be seen during the operation, but may be delayed and seen during the period of intensive care after the operation. Avoidable renal, respiratory and hepatic impairment may all be seen as a consequence of poor pre-operative preparation of a patient.

The morbidity and mortality occurring as a consequence of poor preoperative resuscitation may be seen days or weeks after operation.

Who to resuscitate before operation?

Clearly the teenager with the recently infected thumb does not need resuscitation, while the 70 year old with faecal peritonitis for the last two days does. Our guidelines for who to resuscitate are shown in Table 24.

Peritonitis for more than 24 h
or
Peritonitis for less than 24 h and any three of the following

Age >65 years	Systolic BP <100 mmHg
Heart rate rate > 100 bpm for more than 2 hours	
	Cold mottled peripheries
Respiratory Rate <10 or >30	Temperature <36.5 or >38.5°C
Urine output < 20 mL/h for > 2h	SaO_2 < 90% on air
Laboratory tests	
Hb <10 g/dL	PaO_2 < 10 kPa
Base deficit > 5 mmol/L	Prothrombin time > 25 secs
potassium <3 or >5 mmol/L	White cell count <2 × 10^9/L

Table 24: Identifying patients to optimise before emergency abdominal surgery.

What to aim for?

To answer this question our guidelines are shown below

Warm peripheries	Systolic BP within 10% of normal
Heart rate <120 bpm	Urine output > 1 mL/kg/h
Serum potassium and magnesium normal	Hb >10 g/dL
PaO_2 >10 kPa	Lactate < 5 mmol/L *or* Base deficit < 5 mmol/L

Table 25: What to aim for when optimising patients before emergency abdominal surgery.

When to operate?

Only a small time window for operation exists once a patient has been resuscitated. If this window is missed then the patient will become more unstable and difficult to resuscitate. The risks of surgery and anaesthesia increase dramatically. Operations should not be postponed because of unsociable hours etc.

Once the patient is resuscitated, operate - do not delay.

The role of dopexamine

This drug is an analogue of dopamine. It differs from dopamine in having significant action at the β receptors and no significant direct action at the α receptors, but is similar in having dopaminergic effects. Used as an *adjuvant* to fluid resuscitation current evidence shows it significantly reduces mortality after major abdominal operations. It should be used in low doses (0.5 - 1 μg/kg/min). Its mode of action is not fully known. At these doses it is more likely to act as an anti-inflammatory agent, rather than as a drug that changes cardiovascular variables. Further work is needed to confirm its use. At the moment we start it before operation and continue for 48 h or until the base excess is normal.

Dopexamine *may* be a valuable adjuvant to pre-operative fluid resuscitation.

It should not be used as an excuse not to replenish blood volume during patient resuscitation.

Pre-operative starvation

Maintenance fluids for the period of starvation will be required. Patients who have their bowels prepared for surgery with purgatives and/or enemas may lose large volumes of both fluid and electrolyte in addition to the preoperative fast.

Treatment

Give 1.5 mL/kg/h of balanced electrolyte solution, for example, Hartmann's solution, to replace baseline losses.

Intraoperative Considerations

During surgery and anaesthesia the following need to be considered:
- Correction of any pre-existing deficits
- Continuation of maintenance requirements
- Replacement of ongoing losses.

The following need to be taken into account when determining a suitable fluid regimen.
- Baseline water is required at an hourly rate of 115 mL/h in a 75 kg adult. This is sufficient to account for an insensible loss of 500 - 1000 mL/day and a urine output in excess of 1000 mL/day.

Surgical trauma will increase the amount of fluid required by increasing tissue losses and other sequestration of fluid. This deficit will be manifest in both interstitial and intravascular compartments. In addition replacement is needed to compensate for the fluid loss as a consequence of trauma:
- Minimal surgical trauma - 3-4 mL/kg/h
- Moderate surgical trauma - 5-6 mL/kg/h
- Severe surgical trauma - 7-8 mL/kg/h
- In many US centres these amounts will be given as balanced electrolyte solution as resuscitation of the interstitial space is considered paramount. However, in Europe, colloids may be used. Because these are more effective at maintaining the circulating plasma volume less fluid volume is needed.

The above requirements are met by the following fluid regimen. One litre of balanced electrolyte solution is givern in the first hour of surgery. Further fluids are given at a rate of 300 mL/h increasing to 600 mL/h if surgical trauma is severe. We use a mixture of Hartmanns solution and modified fluid gelatin. Aim to keep urine output > 1 mL/kg/h. If bleeding, give red blood cells to maintain a haematocrit ≈ 30 and use longer acting colloids to replace plasma volume loss.

> If colloids are used to replace the plasma volume losses that will occur because of fluid sequestration, smaller volumes will be needed than if crystalloids are used.

Intraoperative fluid losses may be overt or covert. Operative blood loss may be obvious but is notoriously difficult to measure and is often underestimated. Large volumes may lie undetected in body cavities, on large swabs or under drapes. Large losses of fluid also occur into the gut during laparotomy, particularly where the gut is operated on. There will also be losses into tissues as oedema (so-called third space losses).

AFTER OPERATION

Additional fluid requirements will arise if there has been inadequate replacement in the operating theatre. In practice it is difficult for these to be accounted for after the event by surgical staff on the ward and they are a common cause of problems. In order to minimise this, intraoperative fluid deficits should be corrected as far as possible before the patient leaves the recovery room and careful recording of intraoperative fluid balance including urine output and blood loss is imperative.

Water and electrolytes will be lost both in urine, the volume of which must be measured hourly, and as insensible losses. Losses of fluid will occur into the gut particularly following laparotomy if an ileus is present. Measure nasogastric, faecal and fistulae losses if possible, but these may be only a small part of fluid sequestered. The development of 'third space' oedema usually starts as an intraoperative event but may continue for some time afterwards and account for 'lost' fluid in the postoperative period.

Another cause of postoperative hypovolaemia which may not be obvious to the surgical staff is the limited time course of the plasma volume expansion of colloids administered intraoperatively. Gelatins have a volume expansion effect of 1-4 hours and even starches have a limited duration of action of 4-24 hours. (Chapter 4). Consequently, large deficits in plasma volume, which were well corrected in the recovery room, may reappear several hours later as the effects of these volume expanders diminish.

Volume requirement

After surgery any adult over 60 kg with normal renal function should be given at least 2000 mL/day of fluid. If the surgery is major this will be largely intravenous and depending on the type of surgery, greater volumes may be needed. In adults without major cardiac or renal disease, the aim should be to provide a safe fluid load and leave the body's homeostatic mechanisms to manage the distribution of fluids and the excretion of any excess. An estimate of an appropriate target volume is made by considering a basic volume requirement and then making a number of additions depending on the clinical scenario.

With normal renal function, a urine flow of 1mL/kg/h is desirable and an appropriate target for therapy. This determines the estimate of the basic fluid requirement. So an 80 kg man should pass 80 mL/h of urine. In making daily plans it is arithmetically easier to think of a day as 25 hours. The same man will need at least 80 × 25 ml, or 2000 mL, a day. It is better to be slightly generous and round up the estimate to a convenient number. Further additions are needed to assess the final daily requirement.

Pyrexia and insensible loss

Insensible loss is water lost by sweating and breathing. The volume loss is about 50 mL/h, or 1200 mL/day. From this is subtracted the volume of water created by the body's metabolism of nutrients, leaving about 20 mL/h or 500 mL/day to be replaced. This will be increased if the patient has a fever or in a hot environment. The increase should be 500 mL/day for every °C over 37°C.

'Third space' losses

With major tissue trauma, local oedema forms (see Chapter 1). This oedema is an explanation for the measured phenomenon associated with major trauma when fluid accumulates in a non-exchangeable compartment within the interstitial space. This has been called the 'third space'. It is a significant volume in major surgery involving laparotomy or thoracotomy. It must also be remembered in soft tissue injuries with major trauma. At least 40 mL/h or 1000 mL must be added only on the day of surgery or trauma to compensate for this.

Gastrointestinal losses

Gastric losses will be revealed if there is a well placed nasogastric tube. Complete outflow obstruction leads to losses exceeding 3 L/day. When no nasogastric drainage is occurring, a prolonged ileus leads to sequestration of similar volumes in the gut. No reasonable estimate can be made, and the proposed fluid regimen will cope with early occult losses. On subsequent days these losses are best managed by adding further fluids in response to the monitoring for signs of hypovolaemia as described below.

Bleeding (see Chapter 6)
Bleeding should be replaced by colloid infusion in the first instance. Where the loss can be measured, such as in drainage bottles, this can guide replacement plans. More usually the losses remain within the body, or are unmeasurable, for example: staining of dressings and bed linen. Repeated estimates of haemoglobin should be made since blood transfusion will be needed to keep the level above 8 g/dL. Haemodilution by the colloid infusion will decrease the haemoglobin level below where it will later stabilise, so that a target of 8 g/dL will suffice in most patients. The target should be raised to to 10 g/dL in patients with cardio-respiratory or cerebrovascular disease.

In the patient with major blood loss, space should be left in any fluid plan for the administration of fresh frozen plasma, cryoprecipitate, platelet concentrates, antifibrinolytics or other promoters of coagulation. (See also Chapter 6.)

Polyuria
Fluid intake must be increased to match urinary loss if it is obligatory as in some forms of renal failure. In general, urine volumes up to 150 mL/h are considered an advantage after surgery since there will be a large excretory load of protein and drug metabolites. Fluid input should increase to allow a high urine flow to continue.

How much fluid?
Fluids are often prescribed on an hourly basis and it is easier to think of giving an hourly rate based on the weight of the patient in kilograms. These calculations of hourly fluid intake assume the patient has been adequately transfused during surgery - if not resuscitate the patient first.

Calculate fluid needs as follows:-

1. basic fluid requirement – 25 mL/kg/day – approx 2000 mL/day
2. insensible loss – 20 mL/h – 500 mL/day
3. pyrexia, add 10 mL/h or 250mL/day for each °C above 37°C
4. anticipated ileus, add 20 mL/h or 500mL on first day only
5. third space loss with laparotomy or thoracotomy, add at least 40 mL/h or 1000mL on first day only
6. any other measurable losses

For more information see Table 26.

	Day	Hourly
Basic requirement	25 mL/kg	1 mL/kg/h
Insensible loss	500 mL	20 mL/h
Pyrexia	250 mL/°C	10 mL/h/°C
Laparotomy or thoracotomy third space	1000 mL on first day only	40 mL/h on first day only
Potential ileus	500 mL on first day only	20 mL/h on first day only
Blood loss	?	?
Measured gastrointestinal loss	?	?
Any other losses	?	?
Total		

Table 26: Plan for fluid needs in a 70 kg adult without pre-existing disease after operation.

Electrolyte requirement

Sodium

Sodium requirements are classically 1 mmol/kg/day. During surgery, most patients will have received 0.9% saline, Hartmann's (Ringer's lactate) or plasma expanders. These all contain at least 131 mmol/L (see Table 6, Chapter 3) and no patient is at risk of absolute sodium deficiency. However, as discussed in chapter 3 solutions made isotonic with sodium can be used for any continuing volume replacement. Sodium rich solutions, rather than predominantly glucose solutions, are more effective at supporting blood volume and remove the risk of water intoxication. Thus if further volume replacement is required, colloid plasma expanders or isotonic saline will be used. A simple guide to the use of solutions after operations is:

- Correction of hypovolaemia is easier done with colloid solutions.
- Planned fluid prescriptions to match anticipated requirements are better done with crystalloid solutions.
- 'Third space' loss is interstitial fluid and replacement with isotonic saline is appropriate.
- Once the circulating volume is stable replacement fluids should be given each day containing sufficient sodium to meet basic requirements. A 5% glucose solution can be given with at least 500 ml 0.9% saline (containing 75 mmol/L) per day. Alternatively, the mixture 4% glucose and 0.18% saline (containing 30 mmol/L) is a convenient solution (commonly known as 'Dextrose saline') to provide the right proportion of sodium in patients who have no additional sodium losses.

Potassium

There is no need to give potassium on the first day after surgery. This is because the intense catabolism induced by surgery will increase extracellular potassium. In addition, renal function cannot be assured and unnecessary potassium could precipitate a hyperkalaemic crisis. However, blood electrolytes should be measured if there is any possibility of hypokalaemia which can lead to muscle weakness and cardiac arrhythmias. Patients after cardiopulmonary bypass and liver transplantation are an exception and potassium supplements are commonly needed in the early hours after surgery. For all patients with normal renal function on subsequent days 0.5-1 mmol/kg/day potassium should be provided. Much larger supplements may be needed in some patients to keep blood potassium between 3.5 and 4.5 mmol/L.

Other electrolytes - calcium, magnesium, phosphate

No specific plan should be made at first for calcium, magnesium or phosphate. Their body pools are large and further supplements are given in response to decreases in blood concentrations. Phosphate commonly needs supplementation. Trace elements and vitamins are required only in prolonged intravenous nutrition programmes.

Compensation for loss of body fluids
The electrolyte content of major body fluids can vary significantly, but the average contents are shown in Table 27. Measured losses should generally be replaced with equal volumes of isotonic saline with appropriate additions of potassium. Note that although gastric contents contain modest amounts of sodium, the chloride content is high which justifies use of isotonic saline for replacement. Large bowel losses such as diarrhoea are a common cause of hypokalaemia, and large supplements may be needed.

	Sodium	Potassium
Basic replacement	1 mmol/kg/day	None first day then 0.5-1 mmol/kg/day

Fluid content average	Sodium mmol/L	Potassium mmol/L
Sweat	60	10
Saliva	60	20
Stomach	60	10
Bile, pancreas	140	5
Small bowel	120	5
Large bowel/ diarrhoea	60	40

Table 27: Estimate for electrolyte requirements in a 70 kg adult without significant pre-existing disease.

Summary
The following guidelines may be useful in patients after surgery:

First 24 hours
- Early priorities are blood and colloid infusions to compensate for blood loss.
- Once blood loss has been controlled, crystalloid infusions begin typically 2000 mL 5% glucose solution with 1000 mL isotonic saline in 24 hours – more if there has been extensive thoracic or abdominal surgery.
- Two litres of intravenous nutrition should be used instead of a crystalloid when there will be a long delay (> 3 days) before eating is likely. The sodium content of the amino acid

solution (often about 70 mmol/L) needs to be remembered when planning any additional crystalloids.
• Potassium supplements are rarely needed at this stage.

Subsequent days
Blood potassium levels should be monitored the day after surgery to establish the need for potassium supplementation. With significant volumes of fluid loss, daily blood electrolytes should be reviewed to ensure deficiencies are quickly corrected. It can be helpful to get sodium and potassium analysis of nasogastric aspirates and fistula losses when these are large. These cations should be given in anticipation of losses, not to replace measured deficiencies. Magnesium, calcium and phosphate should be monitored twice weekly.

Use of colloids
Immediately after surgery, blood volume replacement should be with colloid solutions because it is easier to monitor their effect. A satisfactory circulation can be maintained with less water and sodium load if colloid solutions are used in preference to isotonic saline solutions. An excess load of both will need to be excreted in the recovery phase.

Use of blood products
Where there is major blood loss, aggressive use of fresh frozen plasma, and platelet concentrates is important, and may be justified by routine estimates of coagulation times. Other therapies include cryoprecipitate, antifibrinolytics, and drug infusions such as desmopressin or vasopressin. All fluids must be effectively warmed to body temperature before infusion as cooling impairs platelet aggregation and will delay control of bleeding.

Nutrition
Nutrition is unnecessary and ineffective in the early hours after surgery. However, after a major operation where it can be anticipated that there will be a significant delay (> 3 days) before feeding can begin, it is sensible to start intravenous nutrition as soon as the circulation has become stable. Food is best given via the gut and a change to enteral feeding must be made as soon as possible. Good planning will help early establishment of tube feeding, for instance by establishing a naso-jejunal tube during the course of surgery.

Monitoring

Urine flow

The most important single monitor of adequacy of fluid replacement is the continuing flow of urine. A target of 1 mL/kg/h should be set. If this is not achieved, the need for further fluid is gauged by reviewing the cardiovascular state.

Cardiovascular measurements

These are described in the section on shock.

Blood electrolytes

Sodium

Routine laboratory measurement is no guide to early fluid requirements after surgery. Hyponatraemia usually indicates water excess, associated with water retention by the kidney caused by excess antidiuretic hormone. Extra sodium infusion is not appropriate. The patient is often oedematous and diuretic therapy and limited fluid volume input may be useful.

Hypernatraemia is normally a sign of dehydration (Page 19). Fluid intake should be increased somewhat but care should be taken not to correct this figure too quickly by infusion of large volumes of glucose solutions as sudden falls in plasma osmolality will ensue. Cerebral damage including central pontine myelinolysis can occur (see Page 17).

Potassium

This is an important measurement after surgery as the need for potassium supplementation can vary widely and unpredictably in the severely ill patient. Rapid increases in potassium will occur in renal impairment and in severe acidosis as with major tissue ischaemia. Decreases will follow major fluid losses - e.g. renal diuresis, or gastrointestinal losses. Insulin given to control hyperglycaemia also causes a decrease. Supplements are best given as bolus infusions of 10 mmol/h (40 mmol over 4h is the usual dose). This may be added to the maintenance fluids, or given as separate more concentrated solution using a controller with repeat potassium estimation to determine further need. Where losses are moderate, additional potassium is added to the intravenous crystalloid infusion.

> The concentration of potassium in iv fluids should never exceed 20 mmol/L unless the infusion is being given through a controller.

Urea and creatinine

Urea production increases in the patient after surgery when catabolic hormones enhance protein breakdown. Usually renal function is adequate to excrete this urea load. Renal impairment will cause an increase in urea and creatinine. Where the urea increases without a concomitant increase in creatinine, dehydration is present and more fluid must be given. An increase in urea greater than 6 mmol/day suggests complete renal failure together with a state of enhanced catabolism.

Calcium and magnesium

There are large body pools of these cations and supplements are not usually necessary early after surgery. Where major body fluid losses occur, supplementation may be required.

Phosphate

Hypophosphataemia is quite common in the severely ill patient. It may cause muscle weakness but its clinical significance remains unclear. Supplements of sodium or potassium phosphate should be given if concentration decreases below 0.8 mmol/L.

Patient weight

Daily weighing is helpful to determine water balance in the patient with a longer term problem. Each weighing must be done with care if it is to be of any value.

Managing the oliguric patient

This is discussed in Chapter 7.

Improving renal perfusion

Urine production should exceed 1 mL/kg/h in the patient after surgery. If it falls below this, a simple protocol should be instituted as illustrated in Figure 18. The principle is to give a fluid challenge and review the effect on cardiac 'filling' pressures (CVP or PAOP). If this fails to correct the oliguria, fluid infusion is continued until reaching target levels of CVP (usually >13 mmHg) or PAOP (usually 15 mmHg). A renal vasodilator should be started e.g. dopamine (2 µg/kg/min) or dopexamine (2 µg/kg/min). Arterial pressure is then reviewed and treatment given as appropriate to increase the pressure to a level likely to be associated with adequate renal perfusion (usually >100 mmHg systolic) but higher in patients who are normally hypertensive. If all these parameters have been met, further fluid challenge may prove dangerous, and fluid administration should be restricted to replacing known losses.

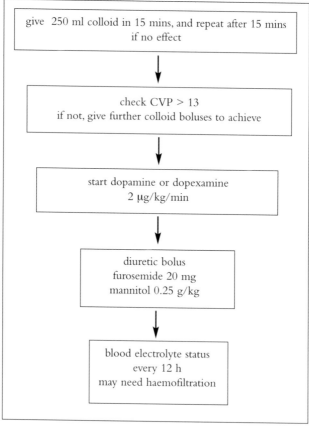

Figure 18: Flow diagram of management of oliguria after surgery.

Diuretics

Once the cardiovascular targets for renal perfusion have been achieved, diuretics should be given to assist clearance of metabolites, and, if there is no urine yet, to confirm that some renal function remains. Suitable diuretics include furosemide 20 mg or mannitol 0.25 g/kg. Mannitol should be avoided if there has been any over-transfusion (e.g. CVP > 17, PAOP > 20). Where urine volumes remain poor despite adequate fluid correction, infusion of furosemide up to 10 mg/h may be useful.

Managing the fluid overloaded

Where fluid therapy has proved to be excessive, mannitol should be avoided and at least 100 mg of furosemide (up to 250 mg may be given in 24 hours) should be given. If this fails to start a diuresis, continuing fluid losses from the patient may restore a safe balance, otherwise the patient will need to be transferred to an intensive care area for dialysis or haemofiltration. The patient will be at risk of developing pulmonary oedema.

Managing the patient with renal disease

Where there is known to be renal impairment before surgery, it is important to establish the normal daily urine volume of the patient. This will form the 'basic requirement' on which other calculations will be made. Reliance cannot be placed on the hourly urine output, and such patients will need early close cardiovascular monitoring after major surgery with careful maintenance of 'filling' pressures.

Managing the patient with cardiac impairment

The recommended fluid intake levels can lead to fluid overload when renal perfusion is poor as a result of cardiac impairment. The normal principles of fluid management are used with care. Pulmonary artery catheter studies (Page 51) may help to give closer control of cardiovascular performance in patients where impairment is significant.

THEORY

Stress response to surgery and renal function

After surgery there is increased secretion of catabolic hormones, such as catecholamines and cortisol, together with a concomitant decrease in anabolic hormones, such as testosterone. This early phase is related to the extent of pain and tissue trauma and is probably triggered by release of cytokines. No single cytokine has been identified, though interleukin-6 levels correlate well with the apparent trauma of surgery. Other important cytokines may be interleukin 1 and tumour necrosis factor α. The duration of the response is prolonged by sepsis, shock and tissue necrosis.

The main hormones that affect renal function are renin, aldosterone and vasopressin. These, too, are increased after surgery. In addition to any specific stimulus from stress itself, there are often factors associated with major surgery that will trigger secretion of these hormones by normal physiological mechanisms. There remains debate over how much of the stress response to surgery is obligatory, and by how much it can be influenced by adjustment of sodium and water input. Water and sodium retention are always present - 60% of a sodium load is retained for at least 48 hours following uncomplicated abdominal surgery.

Renin

Renin levels increase in response to any decrease in renal perfusion that is a common association with major surgery. Stimuli in the afferent arteriole arise from decrease in wall tension, from increased sympathetic tone to the arteriole's granular cells (which produce the renin), and from any change in sodium load at the adjacent macula densa. However, even where the circulation is stable, renin levels increase after surgery. The influence of renin is shown in Figure 19.

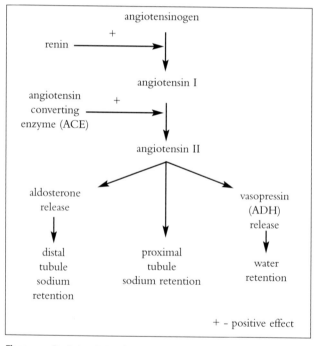

Figure 19: Renin-angiotensin system.

Vasopressin

Vasopressin is a neural hormone secreted by the posterior pituitary gland in response to a variety of stimuli shown in Table 28

1.	Increased plasma osmolality
2.	Decreased blood volume
3.	Angiotensin II
4.	Pain, emotion, stress
5.	Drugs including morphine

Table 28: Stimuli causing secretion of vasopressin.

Vasopressin levels always increase in association with surgery. It acts on V2 receptors in the collecting ducts to increase cyclic AMP that promotes permeability to water. The water passes into the hypertonic interstitium – the urine becomes more concentrated and the body osmolality will decrease.

Abnormalities of vasopressin excretion are described on Page 20.

Aldosterone

Aldosterone levels are also high following surgery that is one of the stimuli (Table 29) to the adrenal cortex.

Aldosterone secretion stimuli
1. Surgery, trauma, haemorrhage
2. Anxiety
3. Angiotensin II
4. High potassium intake
5. Low sodium intake
6. Right heart failure and any rise in inferior venal caval pressure
7. Standing

Table 29: Stimuli causing secretion of aldosterone.

It has a generalised effect to reduce sodium loss in urine, sweat, saliva and gastric juice. In the kidney it acts on the distal convoluted tubule and the collecting duct. The sodium is exchanged for potassium and hydrogen ions by an ATP dependant transport pump in the epithelial cells so that the urine will be acid and potassium rich.

Children

Introduction

Although the principles of fluid balance in children are the same as in adults there are a number of complicating factors that make life more difficult for the junior doctor. The first is an unfortunate tendency for children to grow! Paediatrics involves looking after children from 3 kg up to 100 kg. Any fluids that need to be given are therefore based on the child's weight or the body surface area. Another important complication is that metabolic requirements, including insensible water loss, vary with age and this must also be taken into consideration.

In this chapter the normal requirements of different age groups of children both in terms of fluid and electrolytes are discussed. Afterwards the unwell child and the evaluation of fluid requirements of re-hydration and volume replacement are described. Finally this chapter will describe the fluid and electrolytes needs of children in the perioperative period.

Normal requirements

The distribution of fluids between compartments is different in adults and children and an understanding of this difference is important in deciding on appropriate volumes and types of fluid to use in children. Although the percentage of bodyweight reflecting intracellular and intravascular fluid is fairly constant at 40% and 4% of total body weight respectively, the infant has approximately one-third of their body weight as interstitial fluid - twice as much as in an adult. Consequently water constitutes about 75% of body weight in infancy, compared to 60% in the adult. This may alter the effects of fluid loss, for example in the physical signs. Thus a reduction in skin turgor (reflecting interstitial fluid) is more readily seen in infants than in adults.

Normal values, physiology or heart rate and blood pressure differ with age. A guide to these is shown in Table 30.

	Heart rate (beats/min)	Systolic blood pressure (mm Hg)
Newborn	120 – 140	55 – 75
1 Year	80 – 100	75 – 85
6 years	70 – 100	85 – 100
Adult	50 – 70	100 – 130

Table 30: heart rate and blood pressure in children of different ages.

Water balance
The new born infant
The rate of growth of the human is never greater than in the first few months of life. It is no surprise therefore, that the metabolic demands of the body, both in terms of nutrition and fluid are greatest during this period. The full term infant requires about 150 mL/kg/day of fluid, although less in the first few days of life- (Table 31). Of this, approximately 30 mL/kg will be accounted for by insensible losses. Normal fluid intake is entirely as milk which provides both fluid and nutrition for the first few months of life. During this period the overall fluid requirement will gradually decrease so that a child at three months will need about 120 mL/kg/day and by the time the infant is one year old the requirements are down to 100 mL/kg/day.

In the pre-term infant fluid requirements are greater than in the term infant. Insensible losses are often much higher with particularly increased loss through the skin. Metabolic demands are also substantially higher. Infants born at less than 35 weeks gestation will often require 180 mL/kg/day and some very pre-term infants can receive up to 200 mL/kg/day for the first few weeks of life, although again this figure is lower over the first days of life.

	Pre-term	Term
Day 1	80	60
Day 3	120	100
Day 7	180	150
3 months	120	
1 year	100	

Table 31: Daily fluid requirements (mL/kg) in the first year of life.

After the first year of life

There are a number of ways of calculating the normal fluid requirements of a child. The simplest of these recognises a decrease in fluid requirements with increasing size. (Table 32). Thus for a 35 kg child, there will be 1000 mL (100 x 10) given for the first 10 kg, 500 mL for the second 10 kg and 300 mL for the subsequent 15 kg, giving 1800 mL in total over the 24 hour period. It should be emphasised that these requirements are based on normal needs and that they frequently need adjustment in disease.

Similarly, the calorie requirement for the same child also works out at 1800 Kcal/24hrs (Table 32).

	Fluid (mL/kg/day)	Calories (Kcal/kg/day)
1st 10 kg	100	100
2nd 10 kg	50	50
Any further kg	20	20

Table 32: Daily fluid and calorie requirements from 1 year.

Electrolytes

These will also vary with age, although not so dramatically as fluid volume. In the infant, immature renal function increases the salt requirements, and 3-4 mmol/kg of sodium and 2-3 mmol/kg of potassium are usually needed daily. In older children this decreases to about 2 mmol/kg/day of each ion. Calcium, magnesium and other ions are broadly given in the same (per kg) dose as in adults. (Table 3). Empirically, approximately 3-5 mmol sodium, and 2-3 mmol of potassium should be given for each 100 mL of fluid. When prescribing additional electrolytes to be added to fluids, care over the concentration (mmol/mL) is essential as it will vary for different ions in the solution.

	Day1-2	Infant	Child
Na^+	0-1	1-3	1-2
K^+	0-1	1-2	1-2
Ca^{++}	0-1	1	1

Table 33: Daily electrolyte requirements (mmol/kg) in children.

Glucose
This is critical, especially in young children. The calorie requirement of infants is approximately 100 Kcal/kg, more than double that in adults. Maintenance of adequate glucose levels in infants is important and hypoglycaemia (even for short periods) can cause permanent brain damage. In infants and small children on intravenous fluids, enough glucose <u>must</u> be given to maintain blood sugar levels.

Dehydrated or septic children may well be hypoglycaemic, and early recognition and treatment is essential. In most settings, 4% glucose 0.18% saline at 3 mL/kg/hr is a sensible addition to other fluids as glucose maintenance.

> Hypoglycaemia occurs quickly in children and may cause brain damage.

The unwell child
Shock
Adequate fluid resuscitation must be given as early as possible. Children are less able to compensate for hypovolaemia than adults as they have less ability to control cardiac stroke volume. They are reliant on an increase in heart rate to compensate for decreasing cardiac output. Children are therefore prone to move quite rapidly

from a state of compensated shock to one where the shock is de-compensated and potentially irreversible. The early recognition of shock in children is therefore of great importance.

The first mechanism used to compensate for a decrease in intravascular volume, whether that is caused by hypovolaemia or by fluid re-distribution (eg. as in septicaemic shock), is to increase the peripheral vascular resistance. This leads to a reduction in blood flow to the peripheries and signs of poor perfusion in the hands and feet. As mentioned earlier, tachycardia is also commonly seen in shocked children, although there are many other reasons for an increased heart rate (Table 34). Evaluation of the unwell child's cardiovascular status must assess peripheral perfusion using colour, temperature and capillary refill of the extremities as well as haemo-dynamic measurements. The time taken to re-perfuse a toe or finger that has been pressed firmly (until it blanches) should be less than two seconds, and similarly the difference between peripheral temperature and central temperature should be less than 2°C. Low blood pressure is seen late in the shocked child.. The presence of hypotension, together with a reduced level of consciousness or poor urine output are markers of severe shock and should prompt immediate and rapid action.

Anxiety
Pain
Fever
β agonists etc.
Shock.

Table 34: Causes of a tachycardia in children.

In the presence of shock, fluids should be given. There remains substantial controversy about whether this should be given as colloid or crystalloid in adults (see Chapter 4). There is even less information in the paediatric literature on which to make an informed decision. Most UK units continue to use a colloid (usually albumin solutions) as their prime resuscitating fluid in sepsis. Boluses should be given in volumes of 20 mL/kg and the patient's response reassessed regularly.

Dehydration

The degree of dehydration in a child may be assessed more easily than an adult (Table 35). Thus for example a child presenting with a history of diarrhoea and or vomiting may be haemodynamically stable but quite dehydrated. This will result in a decreased skin turgor. Picking a small fold of skin between one's fingers and releasing it results in a slow return to normal. The eyes are sunken and in children less than one year old feel the anterior fontanelle which may be depressed if there is substantial dehydration. In these situations assessment of the serum electrolytes is important and the fluid should be prescribed to cover both the normal requirements of the child and to provide re-hydration over 24-48 hours. If the child is severely dehydrated an immediate fluid bolus (20-30 mL/kg) should be given (which is taken off the total replacement needed) and the duration of rehydration increased.

Physiological state	Symptoms	Fluid deficit (mL/kg)
Mild (2.5%)	Thirst, dry mucous membranes	40-50
Moderate (5-10%)	+ mild reduction in skin turgor, tachycardia, reduced urine output	60-90
Severe (>10%)	+ sunken fontanelle and eyeballs, reduced blood pressure, markedly reduced turgor, reduced level of consciousness.	>100

Table 35: Assessment of dehydration in infants.

Replacement is usually given as 0.45% saline with 5% glucose, but will depend on the serum electrolytes.

Be aware that in a small number of very sick infants, there may be an undiagnosed underlying metabolic or cardiac disease. Unexplained collapse, especially with hypoglycaemia and coma, should raise the possibility of metabolic disorders. Glucose should be urgently given and blood and urine saved (and frozen at -70°C) for later analysis. Some cardiac conditions (such as aortic coarctation) can present also, and consideration of this (heart murmur? femoral pulses?) is important.

To illustrate how to deal with these problems a case history is shown below.

A two-month-old baby normally weighing 5 kg presents with a three-day history of diarrhoea and vomiting. She weighs 4.7 kg (approx 6% loss), with a heart rate of 120, mildly reduced skin turgor, a dry mouth and concentrated urine. The fluid deficit is thus approximately 70 mL/kg (of <u>original</u> weight) i.e. 350 mL. (Table 35). In view of the vomiting this is needed as replacement. An initial bolus of fluid is not needed, so the replacement was given over 24 hours at 15 mL/hr, 0.45% saline, 5% glucose. In <u>addition</u>, the normal requirements (120 mL/kg, i.e. 600 mL) are needed. The serum electrolytes were essentially normal, and so were given as 4% glucose, 0.18% saline. A total rate of 15 + 25 = 40 mL/hr will be needed, with regular checks of blood sugar, and 12 hourly electrolytes.

Perioperative care
Care of the infant or child peri-operatively requires special mention. Conditions presenting acutely may require resuscitation and stabilisation before surgery. In pyloric stenosis, for example, severe dehydration and electrolyte disturbance (marked metabolic alkalosis) may be present. This should be assessed and often corrected prior to surgery. Blood sugar should be carefully monitored, both in sick children as well as infants starved before surgery.

Fluid requirements after surgery should always be discussed with the surgeon involved, as they will vary with the surgery and with the findings. In broad terms, fluid restriction to one-third daily requirements on Day 1, two-thirds on Day 2 and full replacement on Day 3 is common practice. In situations where increased loss (especially GI loss) occurs, extra replacement may be needed.

Consideration of the electrolyte content of fluids lost from the body is important (Table 36).

	Na (mmol/L)	K+ (mmol/L)	Cl (mmol/L)
Gastric	20–80	5–20	100–150
Pancreatic	120–140	5–15	90–120
Small intestine	100–140	5–15	90–130
Biliary	120–140	5–15	80–120

Table 36: Electrolyte composition of body fluids.

Summary

Although the principles of fluid balance (careful consideration of volume, solutes and route of administration) remain the same in all age groups, there are important considerations when giving fluids to children. The prescriber must recognise the different physiology of children when assessing them, appreciating the normal heart rates, respiratory rates and blood pressures for different ages. Compensatory mechanisms and therefore clinical findings vary from adult practice and these must be recognised. Finally they must have a scheme for assessing both normal and replacement volumes for different age groups. In all of this, common sense must prevail. Even in small children there is flexibility and homeostasis will often be maintained, as long as renal function is normal. Regular reassessment, clinically and biochemically (never forgetting the glucose!) will guide the sensible clinician safely through!

SUGGESTED FURTHER READING

Chapter 1

Roe, P.G. (1998) Fluid therapy. In: Morgan & Hall, *Short Practice of Anaesthesia*. Chapman & Hall, London.

Worthley, L. (1994) Body fluid spaces. In: *Synopsis of Intensive Care, Medicine*, Chapter 42, Churchill Livingstone, London.

Worthley, L. (1994) Fluid and electrolyte therapy. In: *Synopsis of Intensive Care Medicine*, Chapter 47, Churchill Livingstone, London.

Roe, P.G. (1998) Perioperative fluid management. *Surgery*, **16**: 7, 165-8.

Chapter 2

Haperin, M., & Goldstein, M. (1994) *Fluid, electrolyte and acid base physiology*. W. B. Saunders, Philadelphia.

Worthley, L. (1994) Body fluid spaces. In: *Synopsis of Intensive Care Medicine*, Chapter 42, Churchill Livingstone, London.

Hamilton-Farrell, (1997). Fluid and electrolyte homeostasis. In: Goldhill, O., and Withington, P. *Textbook of Intensive Care*, Chapter 16 Chapman & Hall, London.

Chapter 3

Carrico, C., Canizaro, P,. & Shires, T. (1976) Fluid resuscitation following injury: rationale for the use of balanced salt solutions. *Critical Care Medicine*, **4**: 46-54.

Roe, P.G. (1998), Perioperative fluid management. *Surgery*, **16**:7, 165-8.

Kavanagh, R., Radhakrishnan, D., & Park, G.R. (1995) Crystalloids and colloids in the critically ill patient. *British Journal of Hospital Medicine*, **11**: 62-66.

Stoelting, R., & Miller, R. (1989) Fluid and blood therapy, *Basics of Anaesthesia* (2nd. edn.). Chapter 18, Churchill Livingstone, New York.

Worthley, L. (1994) Fluid and electrolyte therapy.
In: *Synopsis of Intensive Care Medicine*, Chapter 47, Churchill Livingstone, London.

Worthley, L. (1994) IV fluids – colloids and crystalloids.
In: *Synopsis of Intensive Care Medicine*, Chapter 13, Churchill Livingstone, London.

Chapter 4

Akcicek, F., Yalniz, T., Basci, A., Ok, E., & Dorhout Mees, E.J. (1995). Diuretic effect of frusemide in patients with nephrotic syndrome: is it potentiated by intravenous albumin? *British Medical Journal*, **310**: 162-163.

Blunt, M., Nicholson, J., & Park, G.R. (1998). Serum albumin and colloid osmotic pressure in survivors and non-survivors of prolonged critical illness. *Anaesthesia*, **53**: 755-761.

Claes, Y., Van Hemelrijck, J., Van Gerven, M., Arnout, J., Vermylen, J., Weidler, B., & Van Aken, H. (1992). Influence of hydroxyethyl starch on coagulation in patients during the perioperative period. *Anesthesia & Analgesia,* **75:** 24-30.

Choi P. T-L., Yip G., Quinonez G., Cook D.L. (1999) Crystalloids *vs* colloids in fluid resuscitation: A Systematic review. *Critical Care Med,* **27:** 200-210.

Cochrane Injuries Group Albumin Reviewers (1998). Human albumin administration in critically ill patients: systematic review of randomised controlled trials. *British Medical Journal*, **317**: 235-240.

Egli, G.A., Zollinger, A., Seifert, B., Popovic, D., Pasch, T., & Spahn, D.R. (1997). Effect of progressive haemodilution with hydroxyethyl starch, gelatin and albumin on blood coagulation . *British Journal of Anaesthesia,* **78:** 684-689.

Nicholson, J.P., & Park, G.R. (1999). The role of albumin in critical illness. *British Journal of Anaesthesia*, in press.

Ruftmann, T.G., James, M.F., & Viljoen, J.F. (1996). Haemodilution induces a hypercoagulable state. *British Journal of Anaesthesia*, **76:** 412-414.

Saddler, J.M., & Horsey, P.J. (1987). The new generation gelatins. *Anaesthesia*, **42:** 998-1004.

Treib, J., Haass, A., Pindur, G., Grauer, M.T., Wenzel, E., & Schimrigk, K. (1996). All medium weight starches are not the same: influence of the degree of hydroxyethyl substitution of hydroxyethyl starch on plasma volume, hemorrheological conditions and coagulation. *Transfusion*, **36:** 450-455.

Webb, A.R. (1990). The physical properties of plasma substitutes. *Clinical Intensive Care*, **1:** 58-61.

Weinbren, J., & Soni, N. Crystalloids and Colloids. In: Goldhill and Withington. *Textbook of Intensive Care*, Chapter 17, Chapman & Hall, London, 1997.

Worthley, L. (1994) IV fluids - colloids and crystalloids. In: *Synopsis of Intensive Care Medicine*, Chapter 13, Churchill Livingstone, London.

Chapter 5

Carcillo, J.A., & Cunnion, R.E. (1997) Septic shock. *Critical Care Clinics,* **13:** 553-574.

Friedman, G., Silva, E., and Vincent., J.L. (1998) Has the mortality of septic shock changed with time? *Critical Care Medicine,* **26:** 2078-2086.

Hardaway, R.M. (1998) Traumatic and septic shock alias post-trauma critical illness. *British Journal of Surgery,* **85:** 1473-1479.

Ledingham, l., McA., Wright, I.H., and Vincent, J.L. Nimmo, W.S., Rowbotham, D.J., & Smith, G. (1994) Cardiovascular failure: In: *Anaesthesia*, 2nd. ed., Blackwell Scientific Publications. Oxford. pp.1792-1817.

Periti, P., Tonelli, F., & Mini. E, (1998) Selecting antibacterial agents for the control of surgical infection: mini-review. *Journal of Chemotherapy,* **10:** 83-90.

Project Team of the Resuscitation Council (UK) 1999. Emergency medical treatment. *Journal of Accident and Emergency Medicine.***16**: 243-247.

Webb, A.R. (1999) Fluid challenge. In: *Oxford Textbook of Critical Care*, Webb, A.R., Shapira, M.J., Singer, M. and Souter, P.M. (eds). Oxford University Press, Oxford. pp.32-34.

Chapter 6

Ali, M.T., & Ferguson, C. (1997) Massive haemorrhage. In: *Textbook of Intensive Care*. Goldhill, D.R., & Withington, P.S. (eds) Chapman and Hall Medical. London.

Conteras, M.A., (ed) (1998) *ABC of Transfusion*. BMJ Books, London.

Donaldson, M.D.J., Seaman, M., & Park, G.R. (1992) Massive blood transfusion. *British Journal of Anaesthesia,* **69:** 621-630.

Hiippala, S., Replacement of massive blood loss. *Vox Sanguinis 74* Suppl **2**: 399-407, 1998.

Mollison, P.L., Engelfriet, C.D., Contreras, M. (eds) (1997) *Blood Transfusion in Clinical Medicine*. Blackwell Science, Oxford.

Chapter 7

Boyd, O., Grounds, R.M., & Bennett, E.D. (1993). A randomised clinical trial of the effect of deliberate perioperative increase of oxygen delivery on mortality in high-risk surgical patients. *Chest,* **270:** 2699-2707.

Wilson, J., Woods, I., Fawcett, W., Hall, R., Dibb, W., Morris, C., & McManus. (1999). Reducing the risk of major elective surgery: randomised controlled trial of preoperative optimisation of oxygen delivery. *British Medical Journal*, **318**: 1099-1103.

Vander, A.J. (1995) *Renal Physiology* (5th. ed.) McGraw Hill, London.

Chapter 8

Cuthbertson, B.H., Noble, D. W. Dopamine in oliguria. *British Medical Journal,* 1997; **314:** 690-1.

McCrorey, C., Cunningham, A.J. (1997) Low dose dopamine: Will there ever be a scientific rationale? *British Journal of Anaesthesia*, **78:** 350-1.

Bennett, W.M. (1997) Drug nephrotoxicity: an overview. *Renal Failure,* **19:** 221-4.

Farrugia, E. (1998) Drug-induced renal toxicity: diagnosis and prevention. *Hospital Medicine,* **59:** 140-4.

Gelman, S. (1997). Renal protection during surgical stress. *Acta Anaesthesiologica Scandinavia,* Suppl **110**: 43-45.

Slater, M.S., Mullins, R.J. (1998) Rhabdomyolysis and myoglobinuric renal failure in trauma and surgical patients - a review. *Journal of the American College of Surgeons,* **186:** 693-716.

Chapter 9

Forfar J.O. and Arneil G.C. *Textbook of Paediatrics.* Churchill Livingstone, London.

Paediatric Vade Mecum (Hodder and Stoughton)

Advanced Life Support Group. *Advanced Paediatric Life Support.* BMJ Publishing Group, London (1997).

Index